Advanced Schema Therapy Techniques

A Comprehensive Practitioner's Guide to Complex Cases, Modes, and Clinical Innovations

Deva Maloney Ventura

Advanced Schema Therapy Techniques: A Practitioner's Guide to Complex Cases and Innovations

Copyright © 2024 by Deva Maloney Ventura

ISBN: 978-1-7641438-7-5

First Edition: 2025

Isohan Publishing

The information presented in this book is designed for educational and professional development purposes only. This book is intended for use by licensed mental health professionals who have received appropriate training in psychotherapy and psychological assessment. The techniques and interventions described herein should be implemented only by qualified practitioners within the scope of their professional competence and in accordance with applicable ethical guidelines and legal requirements.

The author and publisher make no representations or warranties with respect to the accuracy or completeness of the contents of this work and specifically disclaim all warranties, including without limitation warranties of fitness for a particular purpose. No warranty may be created or extended by sales or promotional materials. The advice and strategies contained herein may not be suitable for every clinical situation. This work is sold with the understanding that neither the author nor the publisher is engaged in rendering legal, medical, or other professional

Table of Contents

Chapter 1: Beyond Basic Schema Therapy

The evolution of schema therapy from its original conception to today's sophisticated clinical practice represents a remarkable journey in psychotherapeutic innovation. For experienced practitioners ready to move beyond foundational techniques, this chapter explores the cutting-edge developments that are transforming how we understand and implement schema therapy with complex cases.

Evolution of Schema Therapy: From 18 Schemas to Expanded Models

Jeffrey Young's original framework of 18 early maladaptive schemas (EMSs) revolutionized our understanding of personality pathology and chronic psychological distress (1). However, contemporary research and clinical practice have pushed these boundaries significantly. Recent theoretical expansions by Arntz and Jacob have proposed additional schemas beyond the original 18, including schemas related to excessive self-sacrifice, status-seeking, and excessive responsibility (2).

The integration of attachment theory has enriched our conceptualization of schema development. Mary Ainsworth's attachment patterns now inform how we understand the formation of specific schema clusters (3). For instance, disorganized attachment frequently correlates with the development of multiple, severe schemas across all five domains, while avoidant attachment patterns often predict schemas in the disconnection and rejection domain.

Contemporary schema mode developments have shifted from viewing modes as fixed states to understanding them as fluid, context-dependent patterns of coping. The work of Lobbestael and colleagues has identified over 20 distinct modes, including culturally specific variations (4). This expansion acknowledges the complexity of human psychological experience beyond the original mode conceptualization.

Case Example 1: Elena's Expanded Schema Profile

Elena, a 42-year-old physician, presented with burnout and relationship difficulties. Traditional assessment revealed high scores on self-sacrifice and unrelenting standards schemas. However, using expanded assessment tools, we identified a previously unrecognized "excessive responsibility" schema that drove her compulsive caretaking of patients beyond professional boundaries. This schema, not captured in the original 18, emerged from cultural expectations in her family of origin where eldest daughters bore responsibility for family wellbeing. Treatment required addressing this culturally-embedded schema alongside traditional interventions.

The experiential turn in schema therapy has brought body-based and creative arts interventions into mainstream practice. Rather than purely cognitive-behavioral approaches, contemporary schema therapy embraces somatic experiencing, expressive arts, and movement-based interventions. This shift recognizes that schemas are not merely cognitive structures but are encoded in procedural memory and bodily responses (5).

Advanced Limited Reparenting Techniques

Limited reparenting remains one of schema therapy's most powerful yet delicate interventions. The process model developed by researchers at the University of Amsterdam provides a structured framework for implementing this technique with precision and safety (6). This model identifies four key phases: assessment of reparenting needs, establishing the reparenting stance, active reparenting interventions, and gradual transition to self-reparenting.

The Positive Reparenting Sequence (PRS) represents a significant advancement in how we conceptualize and deliver reparenting experiences (7). Unlike traditional approaches that focus primarily on meeting unmet childhood needs, PRS emphasizes creating new positive experiences that contradict schema-based predictions. This involves three components:

1. **Anticipatory reparenting** - Helping clients imagine receiving the care they needed
2. **Experiential reparenting** - Providing corrective emotional experiences in session
3. **Integrative reparenting** - Supporting clients in internalizing these experiences

Cultural considerations have become increasingly important in limited reparenting applications. What constitutes appropriate therapeutic warmth, physical contact, or emotional expression varies dramatically across cultures. For example, in collectivist cultures, reparenting often needs to acknowledge family loyalty schemas while still promoting individuation (8).

Case Example 2: James and the Reparenting Boundary Challenge

James, a 38-year-old investment banker with severe emotional deprivation schema, initially responded well to limited reparenting. However, his cultural background (British upper-class) created unique challenges. Direct emotional warmth felt threatening and "unprofessional" to him. We adapted the reparenting approach using metaphors from his world - describing emotional support as "portfolio diversification" and consistent care as "steady returns on emotional investment." This culturally syntonic approach allowed him to accept reparenting while maintaining his sense of dignity.

Boundary management in limited reparenting requires exquisite clinical judgment. The therapist must provide enough corrective

3

experience to heal developmental wounds while maintaining professional boundaries that ensure safety and promote eventual autonomy. Recent guidelines suggest using a "reparenting contract" that explicitly outlines what the therapist will and won't provide, reducing ambiguity and preventing boundary violations (9).

Sophisticated Imagery Rescripting Protocols

Imagery rescripting has evolved from simple single-session interventions to sophisticated multi-session protocols tailored to trauma complexity. Contemporary approaches recognize that different trauma types require different rescripting strategies (10).

The debate between therapist-as-rescuer versus patient-as-rescuer approaches has been resolved through a nuanced understanding of when each is appropriate. Research indicates that therapist-as-rescuer works best in early treatment phases and with severe developmental trauma, while patient-as-rescuer promotes empowerment in later stages (11). Many protocols now use a graduated approach:

- **Sessions 1-3**: Therapist enters as powerful rescuer
- **Sessions 4-6**: Patient's adult self joins therapist in rescue
- **Sessions 7+**: Patient's adult self leads rescue with therapist support

Integration with safe place imagery has become standard practice, providing stabilization before and after rescripting work. The safe place serves as both a preparatory resource and a return point after difficult imagery work. Advanced practitioners now customize safe places to address specific schema needs - for instance, a client with abandonment schema might develop a safe place where consistent, reliable figures are always present (12).

4

Case Example 3: Sarah's Complex Rescue

Sarah, a 45-year-old teacher, suffered repeated sexual abuse from ages 6-10. Her imagery work required a carefully orchestrated multi-session approach. Initial sessions focused on building an elaborate safe place - a mountain cabin with her grandmother (her only safe attachment figure). We then progressed through multiple rescue scenarios:

Session 1: I entered the imagery as a protective figure, stopping the perpetrator and removing young Sarah to safety. Sarah observed from her adult perspective, building tolerance for the imagery.

Session 2: Sarah's adult self joined me in the rescue, initially just standing beside me as I confronted the perpetrator. She comforted her child self while I handled the confrontation.

Session 3: Sarah's adult self took the lead in protecting her child self, with me as backup. She found her voice, setting boundaries with the perpetrator using words she wished she'd had as a child.

Sessions 4-6: We rescripted different abuse memories, with Sarah increasingly taking charge. By session 6, she could enter imagery independently, rescue her child self, and provide self-soothing.

The protocol included specific elements for complex trauma: grounding exercises every 10 minutes, bilateral stimulation during rescripting, and post-session integration work. Sarah's nightmares decreased by 80% and her emotional regulation improved significantly.

Third-Wave Therapy Integration

The integration of third-wave therapies with schema therapy represents a natural evolution, addressing limitations in traditional cognitive-behavioral approaches. Mindfulness-based schema therapy adaptations help clients develop metacognitive awareness of schema activation, creating space between trigger and response (13).

ACT (Acceptance and Commitment Therapy) integration particularly enhances work with avoidance-based coping modes. Rather than challenging schemas directly, ACT-informed schema therapy helps clients notice schemas mindfully while committing to values-based action despite schema activation (14). This approach proves especially helpful with entrenched schemas resistant to traditional cognitive techniques.

The integration process typically involves:

- **Mindful schema awareness**: Teaching clients to notice schema activation with curiosity rather than judgment
- **Values clarification**: Identifying values often obscured by schema-driven behavior
- **Committed action**: Taking steps aligned with values even when schemas are triggered
- **Defusion techniques**: Creating distance from schema-related thoughts without trying to change them

Case Example 4: Marcus and Mindful Schemas

Marcus, a 35-year-old architect, struggled with abandonment schema that created relationship chaos. Traditional challenging of his catastrophic predictions provided limited relief. Integrating ACT principles transformed his treatment:

We began with mindfulness exercises helping Marcus notice physical sensations accompanying schema activation - tightness in chest, shallow breathing, muscle tension. He learned to observe these sensations without immediately acting on abandonment fears.

Values exploration revealed that connection and intimacy mattered deeply to him, yet his schema-driven behaviors (constant reassurance-seeking, jealousy, preemptive rejection) pushed partners away. We used the metaphor of schemas as "old GPS systems" giving outdated directions - he could notice them without following their guidance.

Marcus practiced "commitment despite schemas" - scheduling regular time with friends even when abandonment fears screamed warnings, expressing vulnerability to his partner while acknowledging (not hiding) his fears. He developed a "schema acknowledgment phrase": "My abandonment schema is active right now, and I'm choosing to act from my values instead."

This integration reduced his relationship anxiety by 60% and helped him maintain his first stable relationship in years.

Advanced Experiential Techniques

Multi-chair configurations for complex mode work have revolutionized how we address internal multiplicity. Traditional two-chair work often proves insufficient for clients with multiple competing modes. Advanced configurations might include:

- **The mode council**: 5-6 chairs representing different modes in dialogue
- **Temporal chairs**: Past, present, and future self perspectives
- **The witness chair**: An observing position for developing metacognitive awareness

Embodied approaches recognize that schemas live in the body as much as the mind. Contemporary schema therapy incorporates:

- **Somatic resourcing**: Building body-based coping before schema work

- **Movement-based mode work**: Using physical positioning and gestures to embody modes
- **Breathwork**: Specific breathing patterns for mode shifting
- **Creative arts**: Drawing, music, and drama to access and transform schemas

Group processes in schema therapy have evolved to include peer reparenting - carefully structured experiences where group members provide corrective experiences for each other under therapist guidance. This approach amplifies healing through multiple attachment relationships while maintaining safety through clear protocols (15).

Technology and Innovation

Virtual reality (VR) applications in schema therapy represent the frontier of technological integration. VR allows for controlled exposure to schema triggers and practice of new responses in immersive environments. Current applications include:

- **Virtual rescripting**: Entering childhood memories in VR for enhanced imagery work
- **Mode practice rooms**: VR environments for rehearsing healthy adult mode responses
- **Attachment simulations**: Safe practice of connection in virtual relationships

Digital schema diaries have replaced paper monitoring with sophisticated apps that track:

- Real-time schema activation using smartphone sensors
- Mood and behavior patterns correlated with schema triggers
- Automated prompts for healthy mode activation
- Progress visualization to enhance motivation

Neurobiological marker integration brings precision to schema assessment and treatment. EEG patterns can now identify schema activation, while heart rate variability biofeedback helps clients recognize and interrupt maladaptive patterns. Some clinics use functional near-infrared spectroscopy (fNIRS) to show clients real-time brain activation during schema work, enhancing metacognitive awareness (16).

Case Example 5: David's VR-Enhanced Treatment

David, a combat veteran with severe mistrust/abuse schema, couldn't engage in traditional imagery work due to hypervigilance. VR technology transformed his treatment:

We began with VR relaxation environments, helping him experience safety. Gradually, we introduced mild trust challenges in VR - accepting help from virtual figures, allowing vulnerability in controlled scenarios. The gamification elements (earning "trust points") engaged his competitive side while reducing threat perception.

For rescripting work, we created a virtual version of his childhood home where he could practice protecting his younger self from his abusive father. The ability to pause, rewind, and retry scenarios gave him control traditional imagery couldn't provide. David reported: "Seeing it in VR made it real but manageable - I could finally face it without drowning."

His mistrust scores decreased by 70% over 6 months, with improvements generalizing to real-world relationships.

Practical Tools for Advanced Practice

The **Limited Reparenting Assessment Scale** helps therapists evaluate:

- Client's reparenting needs across developmental stages

- Cultural factors affecting reparenting receptivity
- Boundary requirements for safe reparenting
- Readiness for self-reparenting transition

The **Advanced Imagery Rescripting Protocol Checklist** ensures comprehensive treatment:

- Pre-rescripting stabilization completed
- Safe place established and accessible
- Rescue sequence planned with client input
- Integration activities scheduled
- Progress monitoring tools in place

The **Third-Wave Integration Worksheet** guides systematic integration:

- Current schema-focused interventions mapped
- Mindfulness/ACT elements identified for integration
- Values exploration completed
- Practice exercises designed
- Outcome measures selected

Building Mastery Through Integration

Advanced schema therapy isn't about abandoning foundational principles but rather building upon them with sophistication and nuance. The integration of multiple theoretical frameworks, cutting-edge techniques, and technological innovations creates a rich therapeutic approach capable of addressing the most complex presentations.

Successful advanced practice requires:

1. **Theoretical flexibility** - Moving fluidly between models as clinical needs dictate
2. **Technical precision** - Implementing interventions with careful attention to timing and dosage

3. **Cultural humility** - Adapting approaches based on client context
4. **Ethical grounding** - Maintaining boundaries while providing deep therapeutic experiences
5. **Continuous learning** - Staying current with rapidly evolving research and techniques

The cases presented illustrate how advanced techniques can transform treatment outcomes. Sarah's multi-session imagery protocol addressed complex trauma that single-session approaches couldn't touch. Marcus's ACT integration bypassed cognitive rigidity that traditional challenging couldn't penetrate. David's VR-enhanced treatment made the impossible possible through technological innovation.

Key Takeaways

- Schema therapy has evolved beyond the original 18 schemas to include expanded models incorporating attachment theory, experiential approaches, and contemporary mode conceptualizations
- Advanced limited reparenting requires cultural sensitivity, clear boundaries, and systematic progression through the Positive Reparenting Sequence
- Sophisticated imagery rescripting protocols use multi-session approaches with graduated responsibility shifting from therapist-as-rescuer to patient empowerment
- Third-wave therapy integration enhances schema work through mindfulness-based awareness, values clarification, and acceptance of schema activation while pursuing meaningful action
- Experiential techniques including multi-chair configurations, embodied approaches, and peer reparenting multiply healing opportunities
- Technology integration through VR, digital monitoring, and neurobiological markers brings precision and enhanced effectiveness to schema therapy interventions

As we advance into increasingly complex clinical territories, these sophisticated approaches provide the tools necessary for transformative healing. The next chapter explores how these advanced techniques apply specifically to complex trauma presentations, where multiple schemas interact in challenging ways requiring our most skillful interventions.

Chapter 2: Complex Trauma and Multiple Schemas

Complex trauma creates a psychological fingerprint unlike any other clinical presentation. When multiple schemas activate simultaneously, they don't simply add up—they multiply, creating cascading effects that challenge even experienced therapists. Understanding these intricate patterns requires moving beyond single-schema thinking into the dynamic world of schema interactions.

Understanding Schema Chemistry and Interactions

Schema chemistry refers to the magnetic pull between complementary maladaptive patterns in relationships (17). Think of it as psychological puzzle pieces that fit together in destructive ways. When someone with abandonment schema meets someone with emotional deprivation schema, they often experience intense initial attraction followed by painful reenactment of their core wounds.

The theoretical framework for schema interactions suggests three primary patterns (18):

1. **Mutual triggering** - Both partners' schemas activate simultaneously
2. **Compensatory dynamics** - One person's coping mode triggers the other's schema
3. **Reinforcement cycles** - Schemas strengthen each other through repetitive patterns

Schema clusters rarely exist in isolation. Research identifies common groupings that tend to co-occur (19):

- **The vulnerability cluster**: Abandonment, Mistrust/Abuse, Defectiveness/Shame

- **The impaired autonomy cluster**: Dependence, Vulnerability to Harm, Enmeshment
- **The disconnection cluster**: Emotional Deprivation, Social Isolation, Defectiveness

These clusters create reinforcement patterns where one schema's activation increases the likelihood of others firing. For instance, when abandonment schema activates, it often triggers defectiveness beliefs ("They'll leave because I'm not good enough"), which then activates emotional deprivation ("I'll never get the love I need").

Case Example 1: Emma's Complex Web

Emma, a 34-year-old marketing executive, presented with what initially seemed like relationship anxiety. Assessment revealed eight co-occurring schemas creating a complex web of interactions:

Primary schemas:

- Abandonment (severity: 6/6)
- Defectiveness/Shame (severity: 5/6)
- Emotional Deprivation (severity: 5/6)
- Mistrust/Abuse (severity: 4/6)

Secondary schemas:

- Self-Sacrifice (severity: 4/6)
- Unrelenting Standards (severity: 4/6)
- Subjugation (severity: 3/6)
- Approval-Seeking (severity: 3/6)

Emma's schema interactions created a self-perpetuating cycle. Her abandonment fears led to excessive self-sacrifice in relationships. When partners didn't reciprocate equally (triggering emotional deprivation), she interpreted this as

14

evidence of her defectiveness. This activated mistrust, causing her to test partners through increasingly demanding standards. When exhausted partners withdrew, it confirmed her abandonment beliefs, starting the cycle anew.

Treatment required mapping these interactions visually with Emma, helping her see how schemas reinforced each other. We used a "schema web" diagram showing trigger sequences and feedback loops. This metacognitive awareness became the foundation for interrupting automatic patterns.

Relationship schema chemistry manifests in predictable patterns (20). Common pairings include:

- **The pursuer-distancer dance**: Abandonment schema paired with Emotional Inhibition
- **The caretaker-taker dynamic**: Self-Sacrifice with Entitlement
- **The critic-defender pattern**: Unrelenting Standards with Defectiveness/Shame

Multiple Schema Presentations in Complex Trauma

Distinguishing simple from complex trauma shapes our entire treatment approach. Simple trauma typically involves single-incident events in otherwise stable individuals. Complex trauma results from repeated, interpersonal violations during developmental periods, creating pervasive schema development across multiple domains (21).

Complex trauma survivors often show generalized schema elevation patterns—high scores across most or all schemas rather than specific elevations. This reflects the pervasive impact of early relational trauma on core belief formation (22). Instead of developing one or two primary schemas, these individuals develop what I call "schema flooding"—overwhelming activation across multiple domains.

15

Developmental trauma profiles vary based on:

- **Age of onset**: Earlier trauma creates more pervasive schemas
- **Trauma type**: Sexual abuse often creates different patterns than physical abuse
- **Caregiver involvement**: Trauma by caregivers creates more severe schemas
- **Protective factors**: Even one safe relationship can limit schema development

Case Example 2: Marcus's Developmental Layers

Marcus, 28, experienced multiple traumas across development:

- Ages 0-3: Severe neglect (mother with postpartum psychosis)
- Ages 4-8: Physical abuse (stepfather)
- Ages 9-12: Emotional abuse and parentification (caring for younger siblings)
- Ages 13-17: Community violence and peer rejection

This layered trauma created distinct schema patterns for each developmental period:

Early neglect established: Abandonment, Emotional Deprivation, Mistrust/Abuse Physical abuse added: Vulnerability to Harm, Subjugation, Defectiveness/Shame Parentification created: Self-Sacrifice, Unrelenting Standards Adolescent trauma reinforced: Social Isolation, Insufficient Self-Control

Marcus didn't just have schemas—he had archaeological layers of them. Treatment required careful excavation, addressing each layer while maintaining stability. We used a "trauma timeline" overlaid with "schema timeline" to understand which experiences created which beliefs.

Complex PTSD and Schema Therapy Adaptations

Complex PTSD (C-PTSD) requires significant modifications to standard schema therapy protocols. The additional symptoms of C-PTSD—emotional dysregulation, negative self-concept, and interpersonal difficulties—interact with schemas in unique ways (23).

Key adaptations for C-PTSD include:

1. **Extended stabilization phase**: Building affect tolerance before schema work
2. **Titrated exposure**: Approaching traumatic material in smaller doses
3. **Dual awareness cultivation**: Maintaining present-moment awareness during past-focused work
4. **Somatic integration**: Addressing body-based trauma responses alongside cognitive patterns

Integration with trauma-focused approaches enhances schema therapy effectiveness. EMDR can process traumatic memories feeding schemas, while somatic experiencing addresses the body's trauma responses (24). The key is sequencing—stabilization through schema mode work often precedes trauma processing.

Managing dissociation within the schema framework requires recognizing dissociative modes as extreme forms of Detached Protector. These aren't just coping modes but survival modes that protected the psyche during overwhelming trauma. Direct confrontation often increases dissociation; instead, we build connection with the protective function of dissociation before exploring alternatives.

Schema Modes in Complex Trauma

Vulnerable Child variations in complex trauma extend beyond the basic vulnerable child mode. Research identifies several trauma-specific vulnerable child modes (25):

- **The terrified child**: Frozen in traumatic moments
- **The abandoned child**: Eternally waiting for caregivers who never came
- **The contaminated child**: Feeling permanently damaged by abuse
- **The invisible child**: Learned to survive by not existing

Trauma-specific modes protect these vulnerable states:

- **The hypervigilant protector**: Constantly scanning for danger
- **The collapsed protector**: Shutting down all feeling
- **The chaotic protector**: Creating crisis to avoid vulnerability
- **The merged protector**: Losing self to avoid abandonment

Healthy Adult development faces unique challenges in complex trauma. Without positive models, clients struggle to imagine healthy responses. Building Healthy Adult mode requires creative approaches—borrowing from admired figures, fictional characters, or the therapist's modeling until authentic healthy responses develop.

Case Example 3: Sarah's Mode Constellation

Sarah, 41, survived cult abuse from birth to age 18. Her mode constellation included:

Vulnerable modes:

- Terrified Little Sarah (age 4): Frozen during ritual abuse

- Abandoned Sarah (age 7): When parents gave her to cult leaders
- Broken Sarah (age 13): After systematic sexual abuse

Protector modes:

- The Scanner: Hypervigilant protector analyzing all interactions for threat
- The Void: Dissociative protector creating numbness
- The Performer: Compliant protector maintaining perfect facade
- The Rager: Angry protector keeping others at distance

Parent modes:

- The Cult Voice: Internalized cult teachings
- The Condemning Voice: Self-hatred for "allowing" abuse

Initially, Sarah had no accessible Healthy Adult mode. We built it slowly through:

1. Borrowing healthy responses from her therapist
2. Creating an "Wise Woman Sarah" based on qualities she admired
3. Practicing tiny healthy choices in session
4. Gradually expanding healthy responses to daily life

The work took three years, but Sarah developed a robust Healthy Adult who could protect her vulnerable parts and set boundaries with her protectors.

Dissociation and Schema Work

The dissociative modes framework expands traditional schema mode conceptualization. Dissociation isn't simply detachment—it's a complex system of self-states developed for survival (26).

These modes often have their own schemas, coping styles, and developmental ages.

Integration approaches for dissociative presentations include:

1. **Mapping the system**: Understanding all dissociative parts
2. **Building communication**: Creating dialogue between parts
3. **Addressing part-specific schemas**: Each part may have different schemas
4. **Negotiating cooperation**: Parts learning to work together
5. **Gradual integration**: Moving toward cohesive self-experience

Safety and stabilization protocols take precedence with dissociative clients. Before any schema work:

- Establish reliable grounding techniques
- Create internal safe places for all parts
- Build dual awareness skills
- Develop crisis plans for dissociative episodes
- Ensure adequate support systems

Treatment Sequencing and Pacing

The three-phase approach for complex trauma provides essential structure (27):

Phase 1: Safety and Stabilization (3-12 months)

- Establishing therapeutic alliance
- Building affect regulation skills
- Developing grounding techniques
- Creating safety in daily life
- Introducing schema education

Phase 2: Trauma Processing (6-24 months)

- Gradual schema exploration
- Titrated imagery work
- Mode dialogues
- Limited reparenting
- Integration of traumatic material

Phase 3: Integration and Recovery (6-12 months)

- Building life worth living
- Expanding healthy modes
- Relationship development
- Meaning-making
- Relapse prevention

Managing multiple schema activations requires clinical finesse. When several schemas trigger simultaneously, prioritize:

1. Safety schemas first (Vulnerability to Harm)
2. Attachment schemas second (Abandonment, Mistrust)
3. Identity schemas third (Defectiveness)
4. Behavioral schemas last (Insufficient Self-Control)

Building affect tolerance underpins all complex trauma work. Without it, schema work retraumatizes rather than heals. Techniques include:

- Window of tolerance mapping
- Graduated exposure to emotions
- Somatic resourcing
- Bilateral stimulation
- Container techniques

Case Example 4: James and Jessica's Schema Dance

James (45) and Jessica (42) sought couples therapy after escalating conflicts. Assessment revealed interlocking schema chemistry:

James's schemas:

- Emotional Deprivation (5/6)
- Defectiveness/Shame (4/6)
- Social Isolation (4/6)

Jessica's schemas:

- Abandonment (5/6)
- Self-Sacrifice (5/6)
- Subjugation (4/6)

Their "schema dance" followed predictable steps:

1. James withdraws due to defectiveness fears
2. Jessica experiences abandonment activation
3. Jessica self-sacrifices to reconnect
4. James feels smothered, increasing withdrawal
5. Jessica subjugates needs, building resentment
6. Eventual explosion confirms James's defectiveness
7. Cycle repeats with increased intensity

Treatment involved:

- Mapping their dance visually
- Identifying choice points for interruption
- Practicing alternative responses
- Individual schema work
- Couples mode work

The breakthrough came when they could recognize the dance in real-time and choose different steps. James learned to verbalize his need for space without withdrawing. Jessica learned to self-soothe abandonment fears without self-sacrificing.

Practical Tools for Complex Presentations

The **Schema Chemistry Mapping Tool** helps visualize interactive patterns:

- Draw circles for each person's primary schemas
- Use arrows to show triggering sequences
- Color-code for emotional intensity
- Add timeline to show escalation patterns
- Identify intervention points

The **Complex Trauma Schema Assessment** goes beyond standard measures:

- Developmental timeline with trauma markers
- Schema development by age period
- Protective factor identification
- Dissociative screening
- Attachment pattern assessment

The **Dissociation Safety Protocol** ensures treatment safety:

- Grounding technique menu
- Parts mapping worksheet
- Internal communication log
- Crisis plan with specific steps
- Support person contact list

Key Takeaways

- Schema chemistry creates powerful interpersonal dynamics where maladaptive patterns reinforce each other, requiring careful mapping and intervention at specific choice points

- Complex trauma generates multiple co-occurring schemas that interact in cascading patterns, necessitating visual mapping tools and systematic intervention approaches
- C-PTSD adaptations to schema therapy include extended stabilization, titrated exposure, dual awareness cultivation, and integration with trauma-focused approaches
- Trauma-specific vulnerable child modes and protective modes require specialized interventions that honor their protective functions while building alternatives
- Dissociative presentations need modified schema approaches including parts mapping, internal communication building, and part-specific schema work
- The three-phase treatment approach (Safety/Stabilization, Processing, Integration) provides essential structure for complex trauma cases with multiple schema activations
- Affect tolerance building must precede intensive schema work to prevent retraumatization and ensure therapeutic progress

Working with complex trauma and multiple schemas demands our highest clinical skills. Yet within this complexity lies profound opportunity for healing. As clients understand their schema patterns and interactions, they gain power over previously automatic reactions. The next chapter examines how these principles apply to specific personality disorder presentations, where schema patterns create enduring interpersonal challenges requiring specialized adaptations.

Chapter 3: Personality Disorder Applications

Schema therapy's expansion beyond borderline personality disorder represents one of the most significant developments in contemporary personality disorder treatment. While originally developed for BPD, schema therapy now offers sophisticated interventions across all personality disorder clusters, each requiring unique adaptations and clinical strategies.

Beyond Borderline: Schema Therapy Across PDs

The historical journey from BPD-focused treatment to comprehensive personality disorder application began with a simple observation: all personality disorders involve early maladaptive schemas (28). Young's initial work with borderline patients revealed that schema patterns, while most chaotic in BPD, existed across all personality pathology. This recognition sparked systematic research into schema profiles for each personality disorder.

Contemporary research demonstrates distinct schema patterns for different personality disorders, though overlap exists (29). These patterns don't just describe symptoms—they explain the developmental pathways creating enduring personality difficulties. Understanding these differential presentations allows for precise, targeted interventions.

Treatment outcome research shows promising results across personality disorder clusters. A major multicenter trial found schema therapy effective not just for Cluster B disorders but also for avoidant and obsessive-compulsive personality disorders (30). The key lies in adapting techniques to match specific personality dynamics while maintaining schema therapy's core principles.

Case Example 1: Michael's Unexpected Journey

Michael, 52, sought treatment for "communication problems" at work. Initial presentation suggested simple social skills deficits. However, assessment revealed schizoid personality disorder with predominant schemas:

- Social Isolation (6/6)
- Emotional Inhibition (5/6)
- Defectiveness/Shame (4/6)

Unlike borderline presentations with chaotic schema activation, Michael showed consistent, pervasive detachment. His schemas operated like a fortress—keeping others out to prevent anticipated rejection. Traditional cognitive challenging failed because Michael intellectually agreed but felt nothing.

Treatment adaptations included:

- Extended assessment phase to build minimal trust
- Metaphorical language replacing emotional terminology
- Imagery work using science fiction themes (his interest)
- Extremely gradual exposure to connection
- Accepting his need for substantial solitude

After 18 months, Michael could tolerate brief, genuine connections with two colleagues. While never gregarious, he developed capacity for meaningful if limited relationships. Success looked different than with other personality disorders— and that's precisely the point.

Cluster A Personality Disorders

Cluster A personality disorders—schizoid, schizotypal, and paranoid—share themes of oddness and social detachment but require distinct approaches. The predominant schemas often include Social Isolation and Mistrust/Abuse, but their manifestations differ significantly (31).

Schizoid Personality Disorder involves profound detachment without the psychotic features of schizotypal PD. Key schemas include:

- Social Isolation (experienced as preference, not pain)
- Emotional Inhibition (ego-syntonic restriction)
- Detached Self-Soother mode dominance

Adaptations for schizoid PD:

- Respect the protective function of detachment
- Use intellectual rather than emotional language
- Focus on practical life improvements
- Accept limited therapeutic relationship
- Avoid pushing for emotional expression

Schizotypal Personality Disorder adds cognitive-perceptual distortions to social isolation. Additional schemas often include:

- Vulnerability to Harm (magical thinking about dangers)
- Mistrust/Abuse (paranoid ideation)
- Different/Special schema (not in original 18)

Modifications include:

- Reality testing without invalidation
- Exploring schemas behind magical thinking
- Building metacognitive awareness
- Addressing trauma often underlying symptoms
- Medication coordination for severe symptoms

Paranoid Personality Disorder centers on pervasive mistrust making therapeutic alliance challenging. Core schemas:

- Mistrust/Abuse (extreme elevation)
- Defectiveness/Shame (hidden by vigilance)
- Punitiveness (projecting internal critic)

Therapeutic relationship building strategies for paranoid PD:

- Radical transparency about therapeutic process
- Acknowledging the kernel of truth in suspicions
- Avoiding premature schema work
- Building evidence of trustworthiness slowly
- Using behavioral experiments

Case Example 2: David's Paranoid Fortress

David, 46, attended therapy only because his employer mandated it after multiple HR complaints about his "hostile" behavior. He recorded sessions, sat near the door, and initially refused standard assessments ("You'll use them against me").

His mistrust schema operated at maximum intensity. Every neutral interaction got filtered through threat detection. Beneath lay crushing defectiveness beliefs—he expected attacks because he believed he deserved them.

Treatment required extreme patience:

- Months acknowledging his accurate perceptions (people did sometimes talk about him)
- Exploring how hypervigilance both protected and isolated him
- Very gradually examining costs of constant suspicion
- Using his own recorded sessions to reality-test perceptions
- Building one small trust experience at a time

Breakthrough came when David realized his mistrust schema was "like wearing dark sunglasses indoors—everything looks darker than it is." He began experimenting with "taking off the sunglasses" for brief periods with safe people.

Cluster B Beyond Borderline

While borderline personality disorder receives most attention, other Cluster B disorders present unique challenges. Each requires specific modifications while maintaining schema therapy's effectiveness.

Narcissistic Personality Disorder involves a complex interplay between grandiosity and hidden vulnerability. Core schemas include:

- Entitlement/Grandiosity (compensatory)
- Defectiveness/Shame (core, hidden)
- Emotional Deprivation (denied but active)
- Approval-Seeking (disguised as superiority)

The key insight: narcissistic presentation often represents a Self-Aggrandizer coping mode protecting against unbearable shame (32). Direct confrontation of grandiosity typically fails. Instead:

- Build alliance with hidden vulnerability
- Use "limited reparenting" for unseen child
- Gradually connect grandiosity to shame
- Develop genuine self-worth
- Practice empathy through mode work

Antisocial Personality Disorder presents ethical and practical challenges. When present, schemas include:

- Entitlement (without compensatory shame)
- Mistrust/Abuse (justifying exploitation)
- Insufficient Self-Control/Self-Discipline
- Punitiveness (toward others)

Special considerations for antisocial PD (33):

- Assess genuine motivation versus compliance
- Set firm boundaries about acceptable behavior
- Focus on enlightened self-interest
- Address trauma if present (common but hidden)
- Consider group therapy for peer confrontation
- Maintain realistic expectations

Motivational enhancement strategies become essential:

- Connect behavior to personal goals
- Highlight how schemas limit success
- Use functional analysis of costs
- Build capacity for delayed gratification
- Develop victim empathy carefully

Case Example 3: Robert's Hidden Shame

Robert, 38, a successful CEO, sought therapy after his third divorce. He presented with typical narcissistic features—name-dropping, devaluing previous therapists, demanding special treatment. Standard measures showed extreme Entitlement elevation.

Deeper assessment revealed:

- Childhood with narcissistic mother who used him as "trophy child"
- Father who oscillated between absence and criticism
- Core memory: age 7, mother saying "You're only lovable when you're perfect"
- Defectiveness schema: 6/6 (hidden by grandiosity)

Treatment focused on the wounded child beneath the CEO:

- Empathic responses to hidden vulnerability

- Exploring costs of perfectionist facade
- Imagery rescripting of childhood criticism
- Building authentic self-worth
- Practicing vulnerability in safe doses

The turning point: Robert cried during imagery work, then immediately attacked me for "making him weak." I responded: "The little boy who needed comfort wasn't weak—he was alone. And the man protecting him isn't bad—he's scared." This validation of both vulnerability and defense opened genuine therapeutic work.

Cluster C Personality Disorders

Cluster C disorders—avoidant, dependent, and obsessive-compulsive—share anxiety and fearfulness but manifest differently. Schema therapy offers hope for these often-chronic conditions.

Avoidant Personality Disorder involves pervasive patterns of social inhibition. Core schemas:

- Defectiveness/Shame (extreme elevation)
- Social Isolation (self-imposed)
- Failure (expected rejection)
- Subjugation (hiding true self)

Schema triads in avoidant PD create self-reinforcing cycles (34):

1. Defectiveness beliefs lead to social withdrawal
2. Isolation prevents corrective experiences
3. Lack of connection confirms defectiveness

Treatment modifications:

- Very gradual exposure to social situations
- Imagery work before real-world practice

- Building self-compassion
- Addressing shame directly
- Group therapy when ready

Dependent Personality Disorder features excessive need for caretaking. Primary schemas:

- Dependence/Incompetence (core feature)
- Abandonment (driving clinging)
- Failure (without others' help)
- Subjugation (to maintain connections)

Interventions must balance support with autonomy:

- Graduated independence tasks
- Exploring developmental origins
- Building decision-making skills
- Addressing abandonment fears
- Preventing therapist dependence

Obsessive-Compulsive Personality Disorder (distinct from OCD) involves perfectionism and control. Key schemas:

- Unrelenting Standards (extreme)
- Punitiveness (self and others)
- Emotional Inhibition (control emotions)

OCPD requires patience with rigidity:

- Start with behavioral flexibility
- Explore costs of perfectionism
- Address underlying vulnerability fears
- Build tolerance for "good enough"
- Practice emotional expression

Group therapy considerations for Cluster C:

- Homogeneous groups reduce shame
- Peer support powerful for avoidant PD
- Reality testing for dependent PD
- Flexibility practice for OCPD
- Graduated exposure to interpersonal risks

Case Example 4: Maria's Perfectionist Prison

Maria, 41, an accountant, sought help for "stress." Her life operated on rigid schedules, detailed lists, and impossibly high standards. She worked 70-hour weeks, had no close relationships, and experienced chronic anxiety about making mistakes.

Assessment revealed:

- Unrelenting Standards: 6/6
- Punitiveness: 6/6
- Emotional Inhibition: 5/6
- Underlying Defectiveness: 4/6 (hidden by perfectionism)

Maria's schemas created a prison. Perfection protected against criticism, but the standards were impossible, guaranteeing failure and self-punishment. Emotional inhibition prevented stress relief, while hidden defectiveness drove the entire system.

Treatment required delicate pacing:

1. First, mapping the costs of perfectionism (health, relationships, joy)
2. Exploring childhood origins (hypercritical father, conditional love)
3. Behavioral experiments with "good enough"
4. Imagery work rescripting childhood criticism
5. Building self-compassion practices
6. Gradually expressing emotions

Breakthrough moment: Maria submitted a report with a minor error—intentionally. When nothing catastrophic happened, she cried with relief: "I'm still worthwhile even with mistakes." This opened exploration of her human right to imperfection.

Group Schema Therapy for PDs

Group schema therapy for personality disorders combines individual healing with interpersonal learning. The evidence base demonstrates effectiveness across personality disorder types, with some advantages over individual treatment (35).

Groups create unique therapeutic opportunities:

- Multiple reparenting figures
- Real-time interpersonal feedback
- Schema chemistry observation
- Peer modeling of healthy modes
- Reduced stigma and isolation

Managing problematic behaviors requires clear structure:

- Explicit group agreements
- Mode-based understanding of disruptions
- Group involvement in limit-setting
- Individual sessions for crises
- Therapist modeling of healthy responses

Exclusion criteria protect group cohesion:

- Active substance dependence
- Severe antisocial behavior
- Acute psychosis
- Inability to control violence
- Severe therapy-interfering behaviors

Different personality disorders contribute distinct challenges and gifts to groups:

- Borderline members bring emotional intensity and awareness
- Avoidant members model courage in showing up
- Obsessive-compulsive members provide structure
- Dependent members show attachment needs clearly
- Narcissistic members (carefully selected) learn empathy

The key is balancing composition for mutual benefit while maintaining safety and therapeutic focus.

Key Takeaways

- Schema therapy effectiveness extends across all personality disorder clusters with specific adaptations for each presentation's unique features and challenges
- Cluster A disorders require respect for detachment needs, intellectual approaches, and extremely gradual trust-building while addressing core isolation and mistrust schemas
- Narcissistic presentations often mask severe defectiveness/shame schemas requiring empathic connection to hidden vulnerability before addressing grandiosity
- Antisocial personality disorder demands firm boundaries, realistic expectations, and focus on enlightened self-interest when genuine motivation exists
- Cluster C disorders benefit from graduated exposure approaches, shame reduction, and careful balance between support and autonomy promotion
- Group schema therapy offers unique advantages through multiple reparenting experiences, peer feedback, and reduced stigma when carefully composed and managed

- Success metrics vary by personality disorder type—expecting uniform outcomes misses the unique therapeutic goals appropriate to each presentation

The complexity of personality disorders demands sophisticated clinical skills and patience. Yet schema therapy's comprehensive framework offers hope where traditional approaches often fail. The next chapter addresses a universal challenge across all presentations: the therapy-resistant client who challenges our clinical skills and tests our own schemas in the therapeutic relationship.

Chapter 4: The Therapy-Resistant Client

Every experienced therapist knows the sinking feeling when a client responds to carefully crafted interventions with "Yes, but..." or stony silence. Therapy resistance isn't failure—it's information. Understanding resistance through a schema therapy lens transforms frustration into clinical curiosity and opens new pathways for engagement.

Understanding Resistance in Schema Context

Resistance serves a protective function, guarding vulnerable parts from anticipated harm (36). What looks like opposition often represents schemas and modes working exactly as designed—protecting the individual from expected pain based on past experiences. The resistant client isn't being difficult; they're being careful.

Schema activation drives most resistance patterns. When therapy threatens established protective strategies, schemas fire intensively:

- Mistrust/Abuse schema creates suspicion of therapist motives
- Defectiveness/Shame schema fears exposure through vulnerability
- Emotional Deprivation schema expects disappointment
- Subjugation schema resists to avoid being controlled

Therapeutic relationship factors significantly impact resistance levels (37). The therapist's approach either confirms schema predictions or offers corrective experiences. For instance, a directive style may trigger subjugation schemas, while excessive warmth might activate mistrust in those expecting manipulation.

Cultural considerations add another layer. What appears as resistance might reflect cultural values around emotional expression, authority relationships, or individual versus collective focus. A client maintaining emotional reserve might be preserving cultural dignity, not resisting treatment.

Case Example 1: Carlos's Cultural Shield

Carlos, 45, a Mexican-American engineer, attended therapy reluctantly after his physician insisted. He answered questions minimally, avoided eye contact, and repeatedly stated "I don't believe in this psychology stuff."

Initial interpretation suggested detached protector resistance. However, cultural exploration revealed:

- Family values emphasizing emotional strength
- Previous discrimination from healthcare providers
- Concern that therapy meant "weakness"
- Fear of bringing shame to family

His "resistance" protected cultural identity and family honor. Adaptation included:

- Reframing therapy as "strategic planning"
- Emphasizing strength in seeking help
- Incorporating cultural values into treatment
- Using technical language from his field
- Respecting his emotional pacing

Once Carlos felt culturally understood, his "resistance" transformed into careful engagement. He later explained: "I needed to know you wouldn't make me betray who I am."

Schema-Based Analysis of Treatment Resistance

Avoidant and Detached Protector modes represent primary resistance mechanisms. These modes differ in their protective strategies:

Detached Protector creates emotional distance:

- Intellectual discussions without feeling
- Agreement without change
- Missing sessions when vulnerability threatens
- Creating chaos to avoid depth

Avoidant Protector actively evades:

- Changing subjects from painful topics
- Excessive humor or charm
- Creating interpersonal conflict
- Substance use before sessions

Mistrust/Abuse and Defectiveness/Shame dynamics create specific resistance patterns. Mistrust manifests as:

- Testing therapist boundaries
- Searching for hidden agendas
- Misinterpreting neutral comments
- Expecting therapeutic betrayal

Defectiveness/Shame appears as:

- Superficial presentations
- Excessive apologies
- Premature termination when exposed
- Attacking therapist to avoid vulnerability

Assessment strategies for resistance must be collaborative:

1. Name resistance non-judgmentally
2. Explore protective functions together

3. Validate historical need for protection
4. Assess current costs and benefits
5. Negotiate gradual change

Case Example 2: Linda's Testing Dance

Linda, 32, with severe mistrust schema, began therapy with aggressive testing. She:

- Arrived late to see if I'd reject her
- Asked personal questions about my life
- Googled me extensively
- Made hostile comments about therapists
- Canceled when beginning to trust

Rather than interpreting, I acknowledged: "You're checking if I'm safe. That makes sense given your history. What would help you assess my trustworthiness?" This validation surprised her.

We developed explicit "trust experiments":

- I'd predict my responses to scenarios
- She'd test if I followed through
- We'd discuss discrepancies openly
- She could voice suspicions directly
- I'd acknowledge when she caught inconsistencies

This transparent process honored her hypervigilance while building evidence of reliability. After six months of "testing," Linda said: "I still don't fully trust you, but I trust that you're trying to be trustworthy."

Motivational Strategies and Engagement

Motivational Interviewing integration with schema therapy creates powerful synergy for resistant clients (38). MI principles align with schema therapy's collaborative stance while adding specific techniques for ambivalence.

Key MI-schema integration points:

- **Exploring ambivalence** about changing schemas
- **Developing discrepancy** between schemas and values
- **Rolling with resistance** as protective mode expression
- **Supporting self-efficacy** for gradual change

PACE principles (Playfulness, Acceptance, Curiosity, Empathy) particularly help with resistant dynamics (39):

- **Playfulness** disarms protective modes
- **Acceptance** reduces shame-based resistance
- **Curiosity** models non-judgmental exploration
- **Empathy** provides corrective experiences

Paradoxical interventions work when direct approaches fail:

- Prescribing the resistance
- Exploring benefits of not changing
- Predicting therapeutic failure
- Joining protective modes
- Celebrating effective protection

The key is genuine respect for resistance rather than manipulation. Paradox works because it validates the protective system while highlighting costs.

Therapist Schemas and Countertransference

Common therapist schema triggers with resistant clients include:

- **Failure schema**: "I'm not good enough to help"
- **Unrelenting Standards**: "I should break through resistance"

- **Approval-Seeking**: "They must like me to progress"
- **Self-Sacrifice**: "I'll work harder than they do"

These schemas create countertransference patterns:

- Pushing too hard (Unrelenting Standards)
- Giving up too soon (Failure)
- Overaccommodating (Approval-Seeking)
- Burning out (Self-Sacrifice)

Personal therapy and supervision needs intensify with resistant clients. Therapists must:

- Identify activated schemas
- Process emotional reactions
- Develop coping strategies
- Maintain therapeutic boundaries
- Seek consultation for blind spots

Self-assessment tools help monitor therapist schemas:

- Session reaction logs
- Body sensation tracking
- Thought monitoring
- Emotional intensity ratings
- Behavioral urge notation

Case Example 3: My Own Schema Activation

Working with Robert, an entitled, dismissive executive, activated my own schemas intensely. He:

- Questioned my credentials repeatedly
- Made condescending comments
- Compared me unfavorably to previous therapists
- Demanded special scheduling accommodations
- Threatened to report me for "incompetence"

My Defectiveness schema fired: "Maybe I'm not skilled enough." This triggered Unrelenting Standards: "I must prove my competence." I found myself over-preparing, arguing points, and dreading sessions.

Supervision revealed my pattern. My supervisor asked: "What if his devaluing protects his own defectiveness?" This reframe transformed my approach. Instead of proving competence, I became curious about his protection needs.

Next session, when Robert attacked my approach, I responded: "You're working hard to find flaws in me. I wonder what would happen if you couldn't find any?" His face crumpled momentarily before hardening again. We'd found the therapeutic edge.

Rupture and Repair in Schema Therapy

Identifying ruptures through a schema lens reveals predictable patterns (40). Withdrawal ruptures often indicate:

- Subjugation schema activation
- Detached Protector emergence
- Abandonment fears
- Emotional Deprivation expectations

Confrontation ruptures typically signal:

- Mistrust schema firing
- Angry Protector activation
- Entitlement defense
- Punitive Parent emergence

Repair strategies using limited reparenting principles:

1. **Acknowledge the rupture** without defensiveness
2. **Validate the schema** activation

3. **Take appropriate responsibility**
4. **Explore historical parallels**
5. **Negotiate moving forward**
6. **Process the repair** as corrective experience

Building stronger alliances through successful repair:

- Ruptures become opportunities
- Repair provides new template
- Trust deepens through survival
- Schemas update through experience

Specific Techniques for Resistant Clients

Empathic confrontation balances understanding with truth-telling (41):

- Validate the protection
- Name the cost
- Express care about consequences
- Invite collaborative exploration
- Maintain connection throughout

Example: "I understand your Detached Protector works hard to keep you safe from disappointment. AND I see how lonely you feel behind that wall. I care about you too much to pretend the wall isn't costing you connection."

Modified chair work for resistant clients:

- Start with observing positions only
- Use objects instead of chairs
- Write modes instead of speaking
- Therapist demonstrates first
- Build gradually to direct work

Behavioral experiments designed for resistance:

- Small, low-risk tests
- Client designs experiment
- Failure reframed as information
- Success defined minimally
- Process more important than outcome

Case Example 4: David's Fortress

David, 48, exhibited extreme Detached Protector resistance. He attended sessions physically but remained emotionally absent—providing factual updates without feeling, intellectualizing every intervention, maintaining perfect composure.

Traditional approaches failed:

- Chair work: "I don't see the point"
- Imagery: "I can't visualize"
- Emotion focus: "I don't feel anything"

Modified approach honoring his protection:

1. Mapped his "fortress" together—drawing walls, moats, guards
2. Explored fortress effectiveness: "It's perfectly designed for safety"
3. Calculated fortress costs: "But no one can visit"
4. Designed tiny windows: "What if you could see out without others seeing in?"
5. Experimented with one-way mirror: journaling feelings privately
6. Gradually opened shutters: sharing one sentence of feeling per session

Progress was glacial but genuine. After a year, David could express: "I feel sad when I leave here." This single feeling sentence represented monumental fortress modification.

His resistance never fully disappeared but transformed into collaborative caution. We worked with rather than against his protection, honoring its wisdom while expanding possibilities.

Key Takeaways

- Resistance represents protective schema activation, not therapeutic failure, providing valuable information about client fears and needs requiring validation
- Cultural factors significantly influence resistance patterns, requiring therapists to differentiate cultural values from psychological defense mechanisms
- Specific modes like Detached and Avoidant Protectors create predictable resistance patterns that respond to mode-specific interventions
- Therapist schema activation in response to resistance requires ongoing self-monitoring, supervision, and personal therapy to prevent countertransference enactments
- Motivational interviewing principles and PACE approaches integrate effectively with schema therapy for engaging ambivalent clients
- Rupture and repair processes, when handled skillfully, strengthen therapeutic alliance and provide corrective experiences for trust-related schemas
- Modified techniques honoring protective functions while gradually expanding possibilities prove more effective than direct confrontation of resistance

Bridge to Advanced Practice

Working with resistance challenges our clinical skills and personal development. It demands we examine our own schemas while maintaining therapeutic presence. Yet mastering resistance work opens doors to helping those who need us most—clients whose protection systems have kept them from previous therapeutic success.

The journey through complex trauma, personality disorders, and resistance builds toward integration—the sophisticated mode work explored in our next chapter. There, we'll discover how advanced practitioners orchestrate multiple modes simultaneously, creating therapeutic experiences that transform rather than merely treat. The resistant client who learns to trust, the personality disorder that softens, the trauma survivor who finds peace—all require the advanced mode work that awaits.

Chapter 5: Integrating Schema Modes Work

Schema modes represent moment-to-moment emotional states that we all shift between throughout our day. For the advanced practitioner, understanding these shifts—and more importantly, the patterns within them—opens doors to therapeutic transformation that simpler approaches often miss. Mode work isn't just about identifying states; it's about choreographing change within the complex dance of human psychology.

Advanced Mode Work Techniques

Mode mapping and sequencing analysis transforms abstract psychological concepts into visual, trackable patterns that both therapist and client can understand (42). Think of it as creating a GPS system for emotional states—you need to know not just where you are, but where you've been and where you're likely to go next.

The process begins with identifying the client's mode repertoire. Most people operate within 8-12 regular modes, though trauma survivors often show more. Each mode has:

- **Triggers** that activate it
- **Behavioral signatures** that mark its presence
- **Emotional tones** that color experience
- **Exit pathways** to other modes
- **Duration patterns** from seconds to hours

Blended mode work addresses the reality that pure modes rarely exist. People often experience mode combinations like:

- Vulnerable Child + Compliant Surrenderer (scared but trying to please)

- Angry Protector + Punitive Parent (attacking self while attacking others)
- Detached Protector + Happy Child (fun without real connection)

Working with blends requires teasing apart the components while honoring their protective partnership. You can't simply remove one mode—you must understand what function the blend serves.

Default mode recognition reveals baseline states people return to when not actively triggered. Common defaults include:

- **Detached Self-Soother**: emotional numbing as baseline
- **Compliant Surrenderer**: people-pleasing as default
- **Self-Aggrandizer**: grandiosity as home base
- **Healthy Adult**: the therapeutic goal

Case Example 1: Mapping Maria's Mode Maze

Maria, 36, a nurse practitioner, came to therapy for "mood swings" that threatened her career. Initial assessment suggested simple emotional dysregulation. Mode mapping revealed a complex pattern:

Her mode sequence typically followed this pattern:

1. **Demanding Parent** (morning self-criticism about appearance/competence)
2. **Compliant Surrenderer** (overworking to prove worth)
3. **Vulnerable Child** (activated by any perceived criticism)
4. **Angry Protector** (explosive response to protect vulnerable child)
5. **Punitive Parent** (savage self-attack for losing control)
6. **Detached Protector** (emotional shutdown to escape self-punishment)

We created a visual map using colored cards for each mode, with arrows showing typical transitions. Maria could finally see her pattern: "I'm on a hamster wheel of hurt." This metacognitive awareness became the foundation for change.

The breakthrough came when we identified "choice points"—moments where different mode transitions were possible. Between Vulnerable Child and Angry Protector, we found a 3-second window where intervention could redirect to Healthy Adult. Maria learned to recognize her chest tightening (vulnerable child activation) as a cue to pause and breathe, creating space for healthier responses.

Mode Dialogues and Chair Work Variations

Multi-chair configurations expand beyond traditional two-chair work to accommodate complex mode interactions. Standard configurations include:

The Triangle Configuration (three chairs):

- Vulnerable Child
- Protective Mode
- Healthy Adult (developing)

The Square Configuration (four chairs):

- Two conflicting modes
- Observing self
- Wise mind/Healthy Adult

The Circle Configuration (5-6 chairs):

- Full mode constellation
- Empty chair for emerging modes
- Therapist position as guide

Temporal adaptations involve placing chairs to represent past, present, and future versions of modes. This helps clients see mode evolution and possibility for change. For instance:

- Past Angry Child (age 8)
- Current Angry Protector (adult version)
- Future Healthy Protector (goal state)

Cultural adaptations require sensitivity to spatial relationships and authority dynamics. Some considerations:

- Cultures valuing hierarchy may need elevated positions for parent modes
- Collective cultures benefit from family member positions
- Some clients prefer floor cushions to chairs
- Movement-oriented cultures may walk between positions

Group chair work multiplies healing potential through witnessed vulnerability and collective reparenting (43). Groups of 6-8 allow for:

- Simultaneous mode work with peer support
- Role reversals where members play each other's modes
- Collective Healthy Adult development
- Real-time schema chemistry observation

Case Example 2: Ahmad's Cultural Chair Challenge

Ahmad, 28, a Yemeni refugee, struggled with severe PTSD from war exposure. Traditional chair work felt alien—sitting while discussing trauma violated cultural norms about male emotional expression. We adapted:

Instead of chairs, we used prayer rugs positioned to represent different modes:

- **Eastern rug**: His "Warrior Protector" (cultural masculine ideal)
- **Western rug**: His "Terrified Child" (war memories)
- **Northern rug**: His "Faithful Self" (connection to Allah)
- **Southern rug**: His "New Life Adult" (integration goal)
- **Center cushion**: Observer position

Ahmad could stand, sit, or kneel on each rug as felt natural. The configuration honored his need for movement and prayer postures while exploring modes. When discussing vulnerable states, he often knelt in prayer position, making emotional expression feel culturally syntonic.

The breakthrough moment: Ahmad realized his Warrior Protector wasn't protecting his Terrified Child but imprisoning him. In his words: "A true warrior protects the innocent, even the innocent within himself." This cultural reframe allowed mode dialogue that purely Western approaches had failed to achieve.

Forensic and Complex Case Mode Models

Offender mode patterns reveal specific configurations common in forensic populations. Research identifies key modes (44):

The Bully and Attack Mode: Proactive aggression for dominance

- Develops from childhood powerlessness
- Seeks control through intimidation
- Often masks vulnerable states

The Predator Mode: Cold, calculating harm

- Dissociated from empathy
- Plans without emotional interference
- Requires specialized interventions

The Over-Controller Mode: Rigid dominance needs

- Cannot tolerate perceived disrespect
- Violence when control threatened
- Often culturally reinforced

Complex dissociation models expand beyond simple protector modes to include:

- **System controllers**: Parts managing other parts
- **Memory holders**: Containing specific traumas
- **Body parts**: Holding somatic experiences
- **Age-specific parts**: Frozen at trauma times

Co-therapy approaches prove essential for complex cases, offering:

- Modeling of healthy relationship
- Split transference management
- Safety through numbers
- Different expertise areas
- Cultural/gender balance

Case Example 3: Derek's Predator Transformation

Derek, 34, entered therapy as court mandate after sexual offense. He displayed classic Predator Mode characteristics— emotionally flat, calculating, minimizing harm. Traditional empathy-building failed completely.

Co-therapy with male/female team provided breakthrough structure:

- Male therapist connected with his "Power Seeking" mode
- Female therapist carefully approached his hidden "Worthless Child"

- Together, we mapped his mode transition from victim to perpetrator

Derek's mode constellation:

1. **Abandoned Child** (mother's drug addiction)
2. **Enraged Child** (father's violence)
3. **Detached Protector** (survival through numbness)
4. **Predator Mode** (power through victimizing)
5. **Empty** (his term for feeling nothing)

The work took three years, requiring:

- Victim empathy through own vulnerability
- Reconnecting to frozen child states
- Building genuine remorse capacity
- Developing healthy power sources
- Creating internal victim protection

Derek eventually developed what he called his "Guardian mode"—protecting vulnerable others as he wished someone had protected him. While he'll never be unsupervised with children, he now works in victim advocacy, using his understanding of predator psychology to help protect others.

Mode Cycles and Sequences

Cycle identification requires pattern recognition across time. Common cycles include:

The Abandonment-Rage Cycle:

1. Perceived rejection triggers Abandoned Child
2. Angry Protector attacks to prevent further hurt
3. Behavior pushes others away
4. Actual abandonment confirms original fear
5. Punitive Parent attacks for "causing" abandonment

The Perfection-Collapse Cycle:

1. Demanding Parent sets impossible standards
2. Over-Compensator works frantically
3. Human limits create inevitable failure
4. Punitive Parent attacks viciously
5. Detached Protector shuts down
6. Cycle repeats after recovery

Trigger mapping involves tracking:

- Environmental triggers (places, times, seasons)
- Interpersonal triggers (types of people, dynamics)
- Internal triggers (thoughts, body sensations)
- Anniversary triggers (trauma dates)
- Cluster triggers (multiple simultaneous)

Healthy mode cultivation requires more than insight—it needs practice. Methods include:

- Daily Healthy Adult journaling
- Mode check-ins throughout day
- Healthy Adult response rehearsal
- Peer coaching in groups
- Therapist modeling

Research Integration: Arntz and Jacob's Work

The extended needs framework by Arntz and Jacob expands beyond Young's original five core needs to include (45):

- **Fairness**: Being treated justly
- **Coherence**: Life making sense
- **Control**: Appropriate influence over environment
- **Pleasure**: Joy and satisfaction
- **Self-Coherence**: Integrated identity

New schema categories emerging from research:

- **Unfairness**: "Life treats me unjustly"
- **Lack of Coherence**: "Nothing makes sense"
- **Helplessness**: "I have no control"
- **Anhedonia**: "I can't feel pleasure"
- **Identity Confusion**: "I don't know who I am"

Cross-cultural validation reveals both universal and culture-specific patterns:

- Core schemas appear across cultures
- Expression varies significantly
- Some schemas protective in original culture
- Mode manifestations culturally shaped

Integration and Clinical Application

Treatment planning with modes requires:

1. **Phase 1**: Mode identification and mapping
2. **Phase 2**: Building Healthy Adult capacity
3. **Phase 3**: Reworking vulnerable modes
4. **Phase 4**: Transforming protective modes
5. **Phase 5**: Integration and maintenance

Progress monitoring through:

- Mode diary tracking frequency/intensity
- Video review of mode transitions
- Standardized measures (SMI)
- Behavioral markers in daily life
- Relationship quality changes

Supervision guidelines for mode work:

- Regular video review essential

- Supervisor models Healthy Adult
- Parallel process awareness
- Cultural competence development
- Self-care for complex cases

Practical Tools for Mode Mastery

The **Mode Flow Mapping Tool** creates visual representation:

- Central circle for default mode
- Surrounding circles for regular modes
- Arrows showing transition patterns
- Color coding for emotional intensity
- Trigger notes on transition arrows

The **Integrated Mode Assessment Protocol** includes:

- Structured interview for mode identification
- Behavioral observation checklist
- Self-report mode frequency
- Interpersonal mode triggers
- Protective and vulnerable mode balance

The **Mode Dialogue Facilitation Guide** provides:

- Opening statements for each mode
- Transition phrases between modes
- Key questions for mode exploration
- Integration statements
- Safety protocols for intense work

Key Takeaways

- Advanced mode work requires mapping complex patterns including triggers, transitions, duration, and blended states rather than simple mode identification

- Multi-chair configurations expand therapeutic possibilities through spatial representation of temporal, cultural, and complex mode interactions
- Forensic populations display specific mode patterns requiring specialized approaches, co-therapy models, and extended treatment timelines
- Mode cycles create self-perpetuating patterns that require careful identification of choice points for therapeutic interruption
- Arntz and Jacob's theoretical expansions add new need categories and schemas particularly relevant for trauma and cross-cultural work
- Effective mode work integration demands structured treatment planning, consistent progress monitoring, and skilled supervision
- Success requires moving beyond intellectual understanding to embodied practice of Healthy Adult responses in daily life

Moving Forward with Confidence

The complexity of mode work can feel overwhelming initially. Yet within this complexity lies profound simplicity—we're helping people recognize their emotional states, understand their origins, and choose healthier responses. Every client who learns to pause at that choice point between Vulnerable Child and Angry Protector has gained freedom they never imagined possible.

As we prepare to explore cultural adaptations in our next chapter, consider how modes themselves are culturally shaped. The Demanding Parent in one culture might be the Good Citizen in another. Understanding these nuances prepares us for truly culturally responsive schema therapy that honors both universal human needs and cultural specificity.

Chapter 6: Cultural Adaptations

Schema therapy's journey across cultures reveals both its universal relevance and the necessity for thoughtful adaptation. What heals in Manhattan may harm in Mumbai. Understanding cultural nuance doesn't dilute schema therapy—it deepens its reach and effectiveness for our beautifully diverse world.

Schema Therapy Across Cultures

Cross-cultural research findings demonstrate schema therapy's effectiveness across diverse populations while highlighting necessary modifications (46). Studies from Asia, the Middle East, Africa, and Latin America confirm that early maladaptive schemas exist universally, though their expression, meaning, and treatment require cultural calibration.

Cultural challenges in schema therapy implementation include:

- **Individualism assumptions** embedded in original framework
- **Emotional expression norms** varying dramatically
- **Family loyalty conflicts** with individuation goals
- **Authority relationships** affecting therapeutic alliance
- **Religious/spiritual exclusion** from secular model

Yet opportunities abound:

- Schema language provides universal framework
- Mode concept translates across cultures
- Imagery work connects to indigenous practices
- Group formats align with collective values
- Reparenting resonates with extended family systems

Therapist cultural competence demands more than surface knowledge. Required competencies include:

- Deep understanding of client's cultural context
- Awareness of own cultural biases
- Flexibility in technique adaptation
- Collaboration with cultural consultants
- Humility about cultural learning

Case Example 1: Kenji's Subjugation Solution

Kenji, 45, a Japanese executive in New York, sought therapy for "stress." Assessment revealed extreme Subjugation schema—but was it maladaptive? In Japanese culture, prioritizing group harmony (wa) over individual needs represents maturity, not pathology.

Deeper exploration revealed the nuance:

- In Japan, his subjugation felt syntonic and meaningful
- In American workplace, it created exploitation
- With American wife, it caused relationship problems
- With Japanese parents, it maintained connection

We reframed therapy goals: not eliminating subjugation but developing contextual flexibility. Kenji learned to recognize cultural contexts and adjust accordingly:

- High subjugation with Japanese elders (cultural respect)
- Moderate subjugation with Japanese colleagues (professional harmony)
- Balanced assertion with American colleagues (workplace effectiveness)
- Open negotiation with wife (marital satisfaction)

Kenji described this as "changing cultural clothes"—not betraying his culture but adapting to context. His stress reduced dramatically once subjugation became choice rather than compulsion.

Adapting Schemas for Different Contexts

Maladaptive versus adaptive determination requires cultural lens. Schemas considered problematic in individualist cultures may be adaptive elsewhere:

Subjugation: Maladaptive in individualist contexts but potentially adaptive in:

- Hierarchical cultures valuing respect
- Collectivist societies prioritizing harmony
- Religious communities emphasizing submission
- Military/institutional settings

Emotional Inhibition: Problematic in expressive cultures but valued in:

- "Face" cultures avoiding shame
- Professional contexts requiring composure
- Cultures viewing emotional control as strength
- Religious traditions emphasizing equanimity

Self-Sacrifice: Pathological when extreme but culturally syntonic in:

- Cultures valorizing maternal sacrifice
- Religious traditions of service
- Collectivist family systems
- Helping professions

Family schema work adaptations accommodate different family structures:

- **Extended family involvement** in collectivist cultures
- **Gender-separate sessions** in traditional societies
- **Elder consultation** in hierarchical families
- **Community healing** in indigenous populations

Individual versus collective identity creates therapeutic tensions:

- Western schema therapy assumes individual self
- Many cultures prioritize relational self
- Treatment must honor both needs
- Integration rather than replacement

Language and Metaphor Considerations

Culturally relevant metaphor systems enhance understanding. Examples:

American metaphors:

- Schemas as "software bugs"
- Modes as "different hats"
- Therapy as "rewiring"

Chinese metaphors:

- Schemas as "ancestral patterns"
- Modes as "weather systems"
- Therapy as "restoring balance"

Latino metaphors:

- Schemas as "family scripts"
- Modes as "different masks"
- Therapy as "healing the soul"

African metaphors:

- Schemas as "village voices"
- Modes as "spirit possessions"
- Therapy as "cleansing ritual"

Emotional vocabulary variations require careful translation. Many languages lack direct translations for schema therapy concepts:

- No word for "assertiveness" in some Asian languages
- "Boundary" implies rudeness in collective cultures
- "Individual needs" sounds selfish when family-focused
- "Emotional processing" foreign to action-oriented cultures

Interpreter integration demands more than linguistic translation:

- Cultural broker role explaining concepts
- Therapy team member not just translator
- Pre-session briefing on therapeutic goals
- Post-session processing of cultural issues
- Specialized training in mental health interpreting

Case Example 2: Fatima's Family Integration

Fatima, 22, a Somali refugee, presented with severe PTSD and depression. Standard individual therapy failed—she missed sessions, gave minimal responses, seemed to worsen. Cultural consultation revealed the problem: individual therapy violated her cultural healing paradigm.

We restructured treatment:

- Included her aunt (cultural mother) in sessions
- Incorporated Quran verses into imagery work
- Used communal healing metaphors
- Connected schemas to "family curses" concept
- Integrated traditional healing with schema work

Her schemas were reframed culturally:

- Abandonment became "tribal disconnection"

- Mistrust became "war wisdom"
- Emotional deprivation became "drought of the heart"

The breakthrough came during family chair work. Fatima's aunt sat in the "Loving Mother" chair, speaking blessings in Somali while Fatima's Vulnerable Child received comfort. This culturally syntonic reparenting achieved what months of individual work couldn't.

Collectivist vs Individualist Adaptations

Family-centered interventions modify standard protocols significantly:

Assessment phase:

- Family constellation mapping
- Intergenerational schema patterns
- Collective trauma history
- Family role assignments
- Cultural expectation inventory

Intervention adaptations:

- Family mode mapping
- Collective chair work
- Group imagery rescripting
- Family schema psychoeducation
- Intergenerational healing rituals

Group harmony emphasis shifts therapeutic goals:

- From individual assertion to skillful negotiation
- From boundary setting to respectful communication
- From need expression to collaborative solutions
- From independence to interdependence
- From self-focus to family healing

Hierarchical respect requires careful navigation:

- Cannot directly challenge elder authority
- Indirect communication about needs
- Therapist cultural positioning matters
- Face-saving interventions essential
- Progress includes family approval

International Applications

Malaysian applications demonstrate successful cultural integration (47):

- Schema therapy combined with Islamic principles
- Prayer incorporated into imagery work
- Schemas connected to spiritual tests
- Group formats respecting gender separation
- Family involvement normalized

Chinese adaptations show promise (48):

- Emphasis on schema psychoeducation
- Less emotional expression required
- Behavioral change prioritized
- Parent modes connected to filial piety
- Group work utilizing collective support

Singapore's multicultural approach provides model:

- Therapists trained in multiple cultural frameworks
- Flexible protocols for different ethnicities
- Language switching within sessions
- Cultural consultants available
- Outcome measures culturally validated

Indigenous population adaptations require deep collaboration:

- Partnership with traditional healers
- Integration of ceremonial practices
- Land-based healing incorporation
- Collective trauma acknowledgment
- Decolonizing therapy process

Case Example 3: Maria's Mestizaje Integration

Maria, 38, Mexican-American, struggled with identity schemas complicated by cultural marginalization. Neither fully Mexican nor American, she felt perpetually defective. Standard schema therapy felt "too white," while traditional Mexican approaches felt "too traditional."

We developed a "mestizaje" (mixed) approach:

- Schemas explored through "borderland" metaphor
- Modes included "Pocha" (Americanized) and "Mexicana" parts
- Imagery incorporated Day of the Dead traditions
- Reparenting included chosen family concept
- Language switched between English and Spanish

Her Punitive Parent spoke in her father's Spanish criticism. Her Vulnerable Child cried in English learned at school. Her Healthy Adult emerged bilingual, claiming both cultures without apology.

The turning point: creating an altar with photos representing different modes/cultures. She could finally see herself as bridge, not broken. "I'm not half of two things," she realized, "I'm whole in my mixing."

Implementation Guidelines

Cultural assessment protocols should include:

1. **Cultural identity exploration**:
   - Heritage culture(s)
   - Acculturation level
   - Identity conflicts
   - Cultural strengths
   - Marginalization experiences
2. **Healing paradigm assessment**:
   - Cultural beliefs about mental health
   - Traditional healing exposures
   - Family attitudes toward therapy
   - Religious/spiritual frameworks
   - Preferred change mechanisms
3. **Practical considerations**:
   - Language preferences
   - Gender of therapist concerns
   - Family involvement expectations
   - Session structure preferences
   - Cultural calendar considerations

Therapist training for cultural competence:

- Immersion experiences in communities served
- Supervision from cultural experts
- Personal cultural awareness work
- Specific population training
- Ongoing cultural humility development

Program evaluation must assess cultural fit:

- Outcomes by cultural group
- Engagement and dropout patterns
- Cultural acceptability measures
- Community stakeholder feedback
- Iterative program refinement

Practical Tools for Cultural Integration

The **Cultural Adaptation Assessment Protocol** includes:

- Cultural identity mapping exercise
- Healing paradigm inventory
- Family structure assessment
- Communication style preferences
- Religious/spiritual integration needs

The **Cross-Cultural Schema Interview** explores:

- Cultural meaning of each schema
- Adaptive aspects in heritage culture
- Conflicts in current context
- Family schema transmission
- Cultural protective factors

The **Cultural Metaphor Library** provides:

- Culturally specific metaphors by population
- Visual aids for concept explanation
- Traditional stories illustrating schemas
- Cultural mode descriptions
- Integration activity suggestions

Key Takeaways

- Schema therapy's universal principles require cultural calibration to avoid imposing Western individualistic values on collectivist populations
- Schemas considered maladaptive in one culture may be adaptive in another, requiring contextual assessment rather than universal labeling
- Successful cultural adaptation involves deep collaboration with communities, integration of indigenous healing practices, and flexible protocol implementation

- Language and metaphor localization goes beyond translation to finding culturally resonant ways of expressing schema therapy concepts
- Family-centered and group approaches often prove more effective than individual therapy in collectivist cultures
- International applications demonstrate schema therapy's adaptability while highlighting the need for ongoing cultural humility and learning
- Effective cultural adaptation enhances rather than dilutes schema therapy's power by honoring both universal human needs and cultural specificity

The Path of Cultural Humility

Cultural adaptation isn't about perfection—it's about partnership. Every session teaches us something new about human resilience expressed through cultural lens. When we honor culture as strength rather than obstacle, schema therapy becomes truly universal in its healing reach.

Our exploration continues into the technological frontier, where ancient wisdom meets digital innovation. The next chapter examines how virtual reality, artificial intelligence, and digital platforms can extend schema therapy's reach while maintaining its human heart. The future of healing integrates the best of tradition with innovation's promise.

Chapter 7: Technology-Enhanced Interventions

The integration of technology into schema therapy represents not abandonment of human connection but its amplification through digital means. When a client puts on a VR headset and finally confronts their childhood bedroom safely, or when AI helps track schema patterns invisible to conscious awareness, we witness technology serving humanity's oldest need—healing from emotional wounds.

Virtual Reality in Schema Therapy

Immersive imagery rescripting through VR transforms traditional visualization into lived experience (49). Unlike standard imagery where clients must generate mental pictures, VR provides rich, controlled environments for therapeutic work. The technology offers:

- **Consistent environments** unaffected by mood or concentration
- **Controllable intensity** through adjustable settings
- **Measurable responses** via integrated biometrics
- **Repeatable experiences** for practice and mastery
- **Safe exposure** to triggering scenarios

Virtual exposure therapy applications in schema work include:

- Childhood homes for rescripting work
- Social situations for abandonment schemas
- Authority figures for subjugation work
- Crowds for defectiveness exposure
- Medical settings for vulnerability schemas

VR biofeedback integration provides real-time physiological data:

- Heart rate variability during schema activation
- Skin conductance revealing emotional arousal
- Eye tracking showing avoidance patterns
- Breathing patterns indicating distress
- Movement data revealing freeze responses

The combination creates unprecedented therapeutic precision—we see exactly when schemas activate and how interventions affect physiological response.

Case Example 1: Sandra's Virtual Victory

Sandra, 29, with severe abandonment schema, couldn't access childhood memories through traditional imagery. Dissociation protected her from feeling but prevented healing. VR changed everything.

We created virtual recreation of her childhood apartment using her descriptions and Google Street View of her old neighborhood. First sessions involved just walking through the space, building tolerance. Biofeedback showed heart rate spikes near her mother's bedroom—site of abandonment experiences.

Session 4 breakthrough: Sandra entered the virtual bedroom where 6-year-old her waited for mother who was out drinking. In VR, I appeared as protective figure while Sandra watched her heart rate on heads-up display. She could see her nervous system calming as we rescued her younger self.

The power came from embodiment—she physically picked up virtual young Sandra, carried her to safety, spoke comfort. Her words: "I could finally feel little me in my arms. She wasn't just a thought anymore."

We repeated scenarios with variations:

- Different ages of abandonment

71

- Various rescue responses
- Sandra as sole rescuer
- Creating new positive memories

After 12 VR sessions, Sandra's abandonment schema scores dropped 70%. More importantly, she could tolerate real-world separation without panic.

App-Based Schema Monitoring

Real-time tracking systems revolutionize schema awareness through smartphone integration. Modern apps can:

Passive monitoring:

- Movement patterns indicating isolation
- Sleep disruption suggesting activation
- Communication frequency changes
- Location data revealing avoidance
- Screen time indicating coping modes

Active tracking:

- Momentary schema assessments
- Mode check-ins throughout day
- Trigger logging with context
- Coping strategy effectiveness
- Mood and behavior patterns

Intervention prompts deliver support when needed most:

- Schema activation alerts
- Healthy mode reminders
- Coping skill suggestions
- Therapist message delivery
- Peer support activation

Therapist connectivity transforms between-session contact:

- Real-time data dashboard
- Pattern recognition alerts
- Crisis intervention capability
- Homework completion tracking
- Progress visualization

Case Example 2: Marcus's Digital Detective

Marcus, 41, a software engineer, struggled identifying schema triggers. His analytical mind loved data but missed emotional patterns. We implemented comprehensive app-based monitoring:

The app tracked:

- Mood ratings 5x daily
- Schema activation checkboxes
- GPS location patterns
- Heart rate via smartwatch
- Sleep quality metrics
- Social contact frequency

After two weeks, patterns emerged:

- Failure schema spiked before team meetings
- Defectiveness increased after dating app use
- Emotional deprivation correlated with isolation
- Unrelenting standards peaked Sunday nights

The visual dashboard revealed what talk therapy missed. Marcus could see his "schema weather map"—predictable storms and pressure systems. This objective data bypassed his intellectual defenses.

We programmed interventions:

- Pre-meeting self-compassion prompts
- Dating app time limits
- Social contact reminders
- Sunday night relaxation protocols

Marcus engineered his own healing: "I debugged my mental code." His engineering metaphor made schema work accessible and engaging.

Online Schema Therapy Protocols

Virtual chair work adaptations maintain therapeutic power despite physical distance:

Technical setup:

- Multiple camera angles for perspective shifts
- Virtual backgrounds representing modes
- Screen sharing for visual aids
- Breakout rooms for mode work
- Recording for review

Creative adaptations:

- Avatar representations of modes
- Virtual objects as transitional items
- Digital white boarding for mapping
- Music/sounds for mode shifts
- Pet appearances for comfort

Digital imagery work leverages screen-based advantages:

- Screen sharing trauma narratives
- Co-creating visual rescripts
- Using movie clips for inspiration
- Building Pinterest healing boards
- Sharing childhood photos real-time

Group therapy platforms enable new possibilities:

- Participants from diverse locations
- Recorded sessions for review
- Chat support during vulnerable moments
- Breakout rooms for pairs work
- Anonymous participation options

AI-Assisted Interventions

Automated assessment through natural language processing can:

- Analyze therapy transcripts for schema language
- Identify mode shifts in speech patterns
- Track therapeutic alliance markers
- Measure homework compliance
- Predict dropout risk

Personalized recommendations emerge from pattern analysis:

- Optimal intervention timing
- Preferred therapeutic techniques
- Effective metaphors and language
- Productive session topics
- Helpful between-session activities

Natural language processing applications include:

- Chatbot support between sessions
- Practice conversations for social schemas
- Automated thought challenging
- Schema diary analysis
- Crisis text recognition

Case Example 3: Elena's AI Ally

Elena, 35, marketing director, traveled constantly for work. Traditional weekly therapy proved impossible. We developed AI-enhanced protocol:

Components included:

- Daily chat check-ins with AI therapist assistant
- Voice analysis for emotional patterns
- Email analysis for schema language
- Calendar integration for trigger prediction
- Automated intervention suggestions

The AI noticed patterns humans might miss:

- Entitlement language increased before family visits
- Self-sacrifice emails peaked during project launches
- Abandonment fears correlated with specific colleagues
- Approval-seeking varied by recipient status

Our sessions became highly targeted:

- Reviewing AI-identified patterns
- Practicing with triggering scenarios
- Adjusting automated interventions
- Processing deeper meanings
- Planning real-world experiments

Elena appreciated efficiency: "It's like having a therapist who reads all my emails and knows exactly when I need help." The AI couldn't replace human connection but amplified therapeutic impact between sessions.

Telehealth Adaptations

Technology requirements for effective online schema therapy:

Minimum specifications:

- Stable broadband connection
- HD camera for non-verbal cues
- Quality audio equipment
- Large screen for visibility
- Private, quiet space

Optimal additions:

- Multiple monitors for materials
- Ring light for clear visibility
- Ethernet connection for stability
- Backup devices ready
- Tech support available

Clinical adaptations for virtual delivery:

- Extended check-ins for connection
- More frequent summaries
- Visual aids replace physical props
- Explicit process narration
- Modified experiential exercises

Privacy and security considerations:

- HIPAA-compliant platforms only
- End-to-end encryption required
- Recording consent protocols
- Emergency contact verification
- Backup communication plans

Integration and Future Directions

Hybrid treatment models combine best of all worlds:

- In-person for intensive work
- VR for exposure protocols
- Apps for daily monitoring

- Telehealth for maintenance
- AI for pattern recognition

Technology selection criteria should consider:

- Client comfort and capability
- Therapeutic goals alignment
- Cultural appropriateness
- Cost-benefit analysis
- Evidence base support

Ethical considerations demand ongoing attention (50):

- Digital divide creating access barriers
- Privacy in age of data breaches
- Human connection versus efficiency
- Therapist competency requirements
- Informed consent complexity

Practical Tools for Digital Integration

The **Schema VR Protocol Library** includes:

- Childhood home templates
- Social situation scenarios
- Authority figure interactions
- Medical/vulnerability settings
- Safe place environments

The **Personalized Schema App Specifications**:

- Customized tracking metrics
- Individualized intervention prompts
- Personal warning sign algorithms
- Preferred coping reminders
- Progress visualization preferences

The **Telehealth Protocol Manual** provides:

- Platform-specific guidelines
- Troubleshooting decision trees
- Clinical adaptation strategies
- Emergency protocols
- Documentation requirements

Key Takeaways

- Virtual reality transforms imagery rescripting from visualization to embodied experience, providing consistent, controllable, and measurable therapeutic environments
- App-based monitoring reveals schema patterns through passive tracking and active assessment, enabling real-time interventions precisely when needed
- Online delivery adaptations maintain therapeutic effectiveness through creative use of technology while requiring specific technical and clinical modifications
- AI assistance amplifies therapeutic impact through pattern recognition, personalized recommendations, and between-session support without replacing human connection
- Hybrid models combining in-person, virtual, and digital interventions offer maximum flexibility and effectiveness for diverse client needs
- Ethical considerations around access, privacy, and human connection require ongoing attention as technology integration accelerates
- Success depends on matching technology to therapeutic goals and client capabilities rather than using technology for its own sake

Embracing Digital Transformation

Technology in schema therapy isn't about replacing the human heart of healing—it's about extending our reach, precision, and impact. When we embrace these tools thoughtfully, we can offer healing to those who might never walk through our office doors.

As we integrate pixels with presence, algorithms with attunement, we discover that technology serves best when it amplifies rather than replaces human connection. The child rescued in VR still needs real-world comfort. The patterns identified by AI still require human wisdom to understand. The future of schema therapy lives in this integration—ancient wisdom of healing enhanced by modern tools of transformation.

Chapter 8: Group Schema Therapy Mastery

Group schema therapy transforms individual healing into collective transformation. When eight people with personality disorders sit in a circle, something magical happens—not despite their pathology, but because of it. Each person's schemas and modes become mirrors for others, creating a hall of reflections where healing multiplies exponentially.

Advanced Group Protocols

Mixed personality disorder groups require careful orchestration but offer unique therapeutic advantages (51). Unlike diagnosis-specific groups, mixed groups recreate the complexity of real-world relationships. The narcissist learns empathy from the dependent member's vulnerability. The avoidant practices connection with the histrionic's emotional expression. The obsessive-compulsive discovers flexibility through the borderline's fluidity.

Protocol selection depends on group composition:

- **High-functioning mixed groups**: Standard schema therapy protocol with modifications
- **Severe pathology groups**: Extended stabilization phase with co-therapists
- **Gender-specific groups**: Addressing unique developmental experiences
- **Cultural groups**: Integrated traditional healing elements

Trauma-focused protocols layer additional safety structures:

1. **Extended screening**: Ensuring trauma readiness
2. **Psychoeducation emphasis**: Understanding trauma-schema connections

3. **Graduated exposure**: From general to specific traumas
4. **Peer support training**: Members helping members safely
5. **Integration sessions**: Processing between groups

Cultural adaptation protocols honor collective healing traditions while maintaining schema therapy integrity. Modifications include:

- Opening/closing rituals from cultural traditions
- Elder involvement in appropriate cultures
- Gender arrangements respecting cultural norms
- Metaphors drawn from cultural stories
- Food sharing where culturally meaningful

Case Example 1: The Mosaic Group

Our "Mosaic Group" included eight members with different personality disorders:

- Sarah (BPD): Emotional intensity and abandonment fears
- Marcus (NPD): Grandiosity masking shame
- Lin (AVPD): Social withdrawal and defectiveness beliefs
- James (OCPD): Rigidity and unrelenting standards
- Fatima (DPD): Helplessness and need for others
- Robert (PPD): Mistrust and hypervigilance
- Anna (SPD): Detachment and emotional restriction
- Carlos (STPD): Odd beliefs and social anxiety

Initial sessions felt chaotic. Sarah's emotional storms triggered Robert's paranoia. Marcus's superiority activated Lin's shame. James criticized everyone's "lack of structure." But within this chaos lay healing potential.

Session 6 breakthrough: Sarah's abandonment panic activated during break. Instead of fleeing (her pattern), she stayed. Lin, usually silent, said: "I see my own fear in you." This connection stunned both. Marcus, typically dismissive, added: "When you cry, I feel...something." Even his uncertainty marked progress.

We used their differences therapeutically:

- Sarah's emotions helped Anna access feelings
- James's structure contained Sarah's chaos
- Lin's vulnerability challenged Marcus's grandiosity
- Robert's vigilance protected Fatima appropriately
- Carlos's unique perspective normalized difference

By month six, they called themselves "The Misfit Family"— finding belonging through shared dysfunction becoming shared growth.

Managing Multiple Schemas in Group

Schema constellation mapping in groups reveals collective patterns invisible in individual therapy. We map not just personal schemas but group schemas—shared beliefs emerging from member interactions.

Common group schemas include:

- **Group Defectiveness**: "We're the broken ones"
- **Group Mistrust**: "Even here isn't safe"
- **Group Abandonment**: "People always leave"
- **Group Standards**: "We must be perfect clients"

Individual-in-group interventions balance personal work with group cohesion:

- **Spotlight time**: Each member gets focused attention

- **Parallel process**: Working individually while others witness
- **Group resonance**: Connecting personal work to others
- **Vicarious learning**: Growing through observing
- **Collective processing**: Group response to individual work

Contagion management prevents emotional overwhelm:

1. **Affect regulation teaching**: Before deep work
2. **Containment protocols**: For intense emotions
3. **Buddy systems**: Pairs supporting each other
4. **Therapist modeling**: Calm presence in storms
5. **Exit strategies**: Safe ways to step out

Case Example 2: The Domino Effect

During session 12, Tom (BPD) shared childhood abuse details. The group's reaction created cascading activation:

- Janet (PTSD) began dissociating
- Mike (BPD) became agitated, wanting to "fix" Tom
- Susan (DPD) froze, overwhelmed by others' pain
- David (AVPD) started planning escape

I intervened quickly: "Everyone, let's pause. Notice what's happening in your body right now." This grounding interrupted the cascade.

We mapped the contagion visually:

- Tom's vulnerability triggered group abandonment schema
- This activated individual protective modes
- Each person's protection triggered others
- Creating group chaos mode

Understanding the pattern gave control. We developed group protocols:

- Hand signals for overwhelm
- Grounding exercises every 20 minutes
- Check-ins before continuing intense work
- Permission to self-regulate without shame

The group learned to surf emotional waves rather than drowning. Tom later said: "Knowing others felt it too made it bearable. We were drowning together, then swimming together."

Group Dynamics and Schema Chemistry

Schema-based group roles emerge predictably. Unlike traditional group roles (leader, scapegoat, mascot), schema roles reflect early maladaptive patterns:

- **The Sacrificer**: Self-sacrifice schema drives caretaking
- **The Protector**: Angry protector mode defends all vulnerable members
- **The Judge**: Punitive parent mode criticizes group
- **The Ghost**: Detached protector remains invisible
- **The Spark**: Impulsive child ignites conflicts
- **The Pleaser**: Compliant surrenderer keeps peace

Therapeutic group culture consciously counters these patterns:

- Rotating leadership prevents fixed roles
- Direct communication challenges subjugation
- Conflict acceptance reduces compliance
- Vulnerability modeling combats detachment
- Limit setting contains impulsivity

Resistance management in groups requires delicate handling (52). Group resistance patterns include:

- Collective silence protecting group vulnerability
- Scapegoating therapist to maintain cohesion
- Intellectualizing to avoid feeling
- Missing sessions simultaneously
- Creating crisis to avoid depth

Specific Techniques for Group Mode Work

Group mode dialogues multiply perspective-taking exponentially. Techniques include:

The Mode Circle:

- Each member embodies different mode
- Client in center experiences all modes
- Provides 360-degree view of internal world
- Members gain insight playing modes

Mode Sculpturing:

- Physical positioning represents mode relationships
- Distance shows connection/disconnection
- Height indicates power differentials
- Movement demonstrates mode dynamics

Collective Mode Mapping:

- Group creates shared mode map
- Identifies common modes across members
- Builds group healthy adult together
- Celebrates mode diversity

Group imagery work creates shared healing experiences:

- Simultaneous rescripting with peer support
- Collective safe place building
- Group witness to individual imagery

- Shared metaphors emerging naturally

Case Example 3: The Collective Rescue

The women's trauma group decided to attempt collective imagery. All eight had childhood sexual abuse histories but felt stuck in individual work. We created a protocol:

Each woman briefly described her "stuck place"—the abuse scene where rescripting failed. Common elements emerged:

- Feeling alone
- No one coming to help
- Shame about not fighting
- Fear of perpetrator's power

We built collective imagery: "Imagine all eight of your child selves in a large room. The perpetrators are outside, trying to enter. But now, all eight adult selves stand guard together."

The shift was powerful. Maria said: "Little me isn't alone anymore. She has an army." The collective strength allowed individual rescripting:

- Each woman's adult self entered her specific scene
- But brought the group's energy with her
- Perpetrators seemed smaller facing eight protectors
- Child selves felt worthy of protection

This collective approach achieved what individual work couldn't—breaking the isolation that trauma creates through shared strength.

Training and Supervision

ISST (International Society of Schema Therapy) certification requirements for group work include (53):

- 25 hours group-specific training
- 40 hours supervised group leadership
- 20 sessions as group member
- Video review of group work
- Written case conceptualizations

Competency development follows developmental stages:

1. **Observer phase**: Watching experienced leaders
2. **Co-leader phase**: Shared responsibility
3. **Primary leader phase**: With supervision
4. **Independent phase**: Ongoing consultation
5. **Trainer phase**: Teaching others

Supervision models for group work:

- **Live supervision**: Supervisor present or viewing
- **Video review**: Detailed process analysis
- **Group supervision**: Multiple supervisees together
- **Peer supervision**: Experienced leaders consulting
- **Self-supervision**: Systematic self-review

Common supervision themes:

- Managing multiple transferences
- Balancing individual/group needs
- Containing therapist anxiety
- Addressing blind spots
- Maintaining therapeutic frame

Quality Assurance

Treatment fidelity in groups requires systematic monitoring:

- Adherence checklists for each session
- Regular video review sampling
- Member feedback questionnaires

- Supervisor fidelity ratings
- Outcome correlation with adherence

Outcome measurement tools:

- Young Schema Questionnaire (YSQ) group means
- Schema Mode Inventory (SMI) changes
- Group cohesion scales
- Individual goal attainment
- Interpersonal functioning measures

Program evaluation encompasses:

- Retention/dropout analysis
- Critical incident tracking
- Member satisfaction surveys
- Therapist burnout monitoring
- Cost-effectiveness calculation

Practical Tools for Group Excellence

The **Group Protocol Selection Matrix** evaluates:

- Diagnostic mix compatibility
- Severity level matching
- Gender composition effects
- Cultural factor integration
- Therapist skill requirements

The **Group Schema Mapping Tool** visualizes:

- Individual schema profiles
- Group schema intersections
- Schema chemistry predictions
- Change tracking over time
- Intervention planning guide

The **Group Competency Assessment Battery** measures:

- Technical skill execution
- Process management ability
- Crisis intervention capacity
- Cultural sensitivity demonstration
- Therapeutic relationship skills

Key Takeaways

- Mixed personality disorder groups create real-world learning laboratories where different pathologies become therapeutic resources for each other
- Schema constellation mapping reveals group-level patterns requiring intervention beyond individual work
- Managing contagion and group resistance requires proactive protocols and sophisticated intervention skills
- Group mode work techniques multiply healing through collective witnessing, shared strength, and diverse perspectives
- ISST certification requirements ensure competency through systematic training, supervision, and skill demonstration
- Quality assurance through fidelity monitoring, outcome measurement, and program evaluation maintains treatment effectiveness
- Success depends on balancing individual needs with group cohesion while maintaining clear therapeutic framework

The Group as Healing Community

Groups remind us that humans evolved to heal in community. The isolated suffering that creates personality disorders finds its antidote in collective understanding. When the narcissist cries for the avoidant's pain, when the paranoid person trusts the group's care, when the dependent member stands strong for others—we witness transformation that individual therapy alone cannot achieve.

As we turn to couples and family work, we carry this truth: healing happens in relationship. The same schemas that wound in isolation can become bridges to connection when understood and transformed together.

Chapter 9: Couples and Family Applications

Love stories often begin with schema chemistry—that inexplicable pull toward someone who feels perfectly wrong in all the right ways. Understanding how schemas dance together in relationships transforms couples therapy from battlefield negotiation to choreographed healing.

Understanding Schema Chemistry

Mode cycle clash dynamics create predictable relationship patterns where each partner's modes trigger the other's schemas in escalating loops (54). These aren't character flaws but learned dances from childhood, now performed with devastating precision on the relationship stage.

Common mode clashes include:

- **Abandoner-Clinger**: One partner's detached protector activates other's abandoned child
- **Critic-Defender**: Punitive parent mode triggers angry protector response
- **Demander-Withdrawer**: Entitled mode meets detached self-soother
- **Controller-Rebel**: Over-controller mode activates rebellious child

Assessment tools for schema chemistry:

- Joint schema questionnaire completion
- Mode observation during conflict
- Trigger pattern mapping
- Attachment style correlation
- Chemistry attraction analysis

Clinical implications reshape treatment planning:

- Individual schema work before couples work
- Psychoeducation about chemistry patterns
- Developing "pause points" in cycles
- Building healthy adult dialogue skills
- Creating new relationship dances

Case Example 1: Tom and Sarah's Perfect Storm

Tom and Sarah felt like "soulmates" initially—that intense connection that signals schema chemistry. Assessment revealed their interlocking patterns:

Tom's schemas:

- Emotional Deprivation (6/6)
- Mistrust/Abuse (5/6)
- Defectiveness/Shame (4/6)

Sarah's schemas:

- Abandonment (6/6)
- Self-Sacrifice (5/6)
- Approval-Seeking (4/6)

Their dance followed predictable steps:

1. Tom withdraws (emotional deprivation coping)
2. Sarah panics (abandonment triggered)
3. Sarah pursues aggressively (seeking reassurance)
4. Tom feels smothered (mistrust activated)
5. Tom criticizes to create distance
6. Sarah self-sacrifices to regain approval
7. Resentment builds in both
8. Explosion resets cycle

During session 4, we mapped their dance visually using floor positions. They could finally see the pattern: "We're both just scared kids trying not to get hurt again," Sarah realized. "But we're hurting each other trying to protect ourselves," Tom added.

This awareness created choice. We developed interruption strategies:

- Tom states need for space without withdrawing
- Sarah self-soothes abandonment fears
- Both take "schema time-outs"
- Return with healthy adult modes active
- Practice new responses

Couples Schema Therapy Protocols

The three-phase treatment model provides structure for complex work:

Phase 1: Assessment and Education (Sessions 1-6)

- Individual schema assessment
- Joint pattern identification
- Psychoeducation about schemas
- Creating shared language
- Building safety agreements

Phase 2: Change Work (Sessions 7-15)

- Individual schema healing
- Coupled mode dialogues
- Interrupting toxic cycles
- Building healthy responses
- Practicing new patterns

Phase 3: Integration (Sessions 16-20)

- Consolidating changes
- Relapse prevention planning
- Future challenge preparation
- Celebrating growth
- Maintenance strategies

Specific interventions throughout phases:

- **Schema Flip**: Partners explain each other's schemas
- **Mode Interviews**: Speaking from specific modes
- **Empty Chair Work**: Addressing partner's modes
- **Imagery Sharing**: Witnessing childhood origins
- **Reparenting Practice**: Offering what was missing

The 16-20 session framework provides enough time for deep change while maintaining focus. Sessions typically run 90 minutes to allow full cycles completion.

Family Schema Patterns

Multi-generational assessment reveals how schemas transmit through families like psychological DNA. Patterns include:

- Grandmother's abandonment becomes mother's self-sacrifice becomes daughter's subjugation
- Father's mistrust becomes son's emotional inhibition becomes grandson's isolation
- Family emotional deprivation creates multiple attachment disorders

Family mode dynamics show collective patterns:

- Whole families operating in compliant surrenderer
- Punitive parent mode as family culture
- Detached protector as survival strategy
- Angry protector defending family honor

Children's schema development within family systems follows predictable paths:

- Parent schemas create specific environments
- Children develop complementary or reactive schemas
- Sibling positions influence schema formation
- Family traumas affect all members differently

Case Example 2: The Morrison Family Legacy

The Morrison family entered therapy when 16-year-old Jake attempted suicide. Three-generation assessment revealed cascading schemas:

Grandfather (deceased):

- Severe punitiveness and emotional inhibition
- Alcoholism and domestic violence
- Created unsafe family environment

Father Robert (52):

- Mistrust/Abuse: 6/6
- Emotional Inhibition: 6/6
- Punitiveness: 5/6
- Coped through workaholism and control

Mother Linda (49):

- Self-Sacrifice: 6/6
- Subjugation: 5/6
- Emotional Deprivation: 5/6
- Coped through endless caretaking

Son Jake (16):

- Defectiveness/Shame: 6/6

- Social Isolation: 5/6
- Failure: 5/6
- Coped through self-harm and withdrawal

Daughter Emma (14):

- Approval-Seeking: 5/6
- Self-Sacrifice: 4/6
- Unrelenting Standards: 4/6
- Coped through perfectionism

The family operated in interlocking modes:

- Robert's punitive parent triggered Linda's compliant surrenderer
- Linda's self-sacrifice enabled Robert's emotional absence
- Jake absorbed family shame through defectiveness schema
- Emma tried to earn love through perfect behavior

Family therapy revealed their unconscious agreement: "We must never feel or we'll fall apart like Grandpa." This shared schema kept them safe but disconnected.

Intergenerational Transmission

Transmission mechanisms operate through multiple channels (55):

- **Modeling**: Children copying parent coping modes
- **Direct teaching**: "Never trust anyone"
- **Environmental creation**: Chaos breeding hypervigilance
- **Emotional climate**: Criticism fostering defectiveness
- **Attachment disruption**: Creating abandonment schemas

Breaking negative cycles requires:

1. Awareness of transmission patterns
2. Grieving what was passed down
3. Choosing conscious change
4. Practicing new patterns
5. Celebrating cycle breaking

Preventive applications focus on early intervention:

- Parent schema assessment during pregnancy
- Early childhood schema prevention programs
- School-based emotional education
- Family schema therapy for at-risk families
- Community support systems

Specialized Interventions

Chair work adaptations for couples/families:

- **Partner Mode Dialogue**: Each speaks from modes to empty chair
- **Family Sculpture**: Physical positioning showing dynamics
- **Generation Chairs**: Past, present, future family patterns
- **Mode Speed Dating**: Quickly switching between modes
- **Healthy Family Practice**: Rehearsing new dynamics

Family imagery rescripting addresses collective trauma:

- Shared traumatic events rescripted together
- Individual imagery with family witness
- Creating new positive family memories
- Healing ancestral trauma patterns
- Building family safe place

Communication training with schema awareness:

- Recognizing schema activation in real-time

- Using "schema language" during conflict
- Time-outs when modes take over
- Repair protocols post-activation
- Daily mode check-ins

Case Example 3: The Chen Family Transformation

The Chen family, Chinese immigrants, struggled with intergenerational conflict. Traditional parents couldn't understand "westernized" children; children felt suffocated by parental expectations.

Schema assessment revealed cultural complexity:

- Parents: Subjugation schemas (adaptive in China, problematic with assertive American children)
- Children: Entitlement schemas (reactive to parents' subjugation)
- Family: Shared emotional inhibition (cultural value becoming dysfunction)

We used culturally adapted interventions:

Tea Ceremony Chair Work: Using traditional tea service as metaphor:

- Each family member served tea representing their needs
- Others received tea representing understanding
- Empty chair for ancestors' influence
- New tea blend representing family evolution

Three-Generation Imagery:

- Grandparents' China survival stories
- Parents' immigration challenges
- Children's bicultural identity
- Creating integrated family narrative

The breakthrough: Father said in Mandarin, "I control because I fear," then in English, "But fear is not love." This bilingual vulnerability opened new dialogue.

Family homework included:

- Weekly "schema dinners" discussing patterns
- Children teaching parents about American emotional expression
- Parents sharing Chinese wisdom about resilience
- Creating new family traditions honoring both cultures

Outcome Measurement

Couples-specific measures track relational change:

- Relationship satisfaction scales
- Schema activation frequency logs
- Conflict resolution improvements
- Intimacy and trust measures
- Individual growth within relationship

High-conflict adaptations require additional structure:

- Separate sessions initially
- Clear safety agreements
- Conflict de-escalation protocols
- Crisis intervention plans
- Possible contraindications assessment

Cultural considerations in measurement:

- Culturally validated instruments
- Collective vs individual outcome focus
- Extended family involvement in assessment
- Cultural values in relationship satisfaction
- Bilingual assessment options

Practical Tools for Relationship Work

Mode Cycle Clash Cards (56):

- Visual representations of common clashes
- Intervention suggestions for each pattern
- Homework exercises for practice
- Progress tracking templates
- Couple-specific customization

Couples Assessment Protocol includes:

- Individual schema interviews
- Joint interaction observation
- Attachment style measures
- Relationship history mapping
- Chemistry analysis framework

Family Genogram-Schema Integration combines:

- Traditional family mapping
- Schema identification across generations
- Trauma transmission patterns
- Protective factor identification
- Intervention planning guide

Key Takeaways

- Schema chemistry creates intense initial attraction followed by painful patterns as complementary wounds activate each other
- The three-phase couples protocol provides structure for moving from pattern recognition through active change to integration
- Multi-generational assessment reveals schema transmission patterns that affect entire family systems across time

- Breaking intergenerational cycles requires conscious awareness, grieving inherited patterns, and practicing new responses
- Specialized interventions adapt individual techniques for relational contexts while maintaining schema therapy principles
- Cultural considerations significantly impact intervention selection, requiring flexible adaptation of Western-oriented approaches
- Success measurement must encompass both individual schema change and relationship quality improvements

The Legacy of Love

Relationships begun in schema chemistry need not end in schema catastrophe. When couples and families understand their inherited patterns, they gain the power to write new stories. The schemas that brought them together in pain can, with awareness and work, become the foundation for deeper understanding and connection.

Every couple who breaks their cycle, every family that heals its generational wounds, sends ripples through time. Children grow up with secure attachment instead of abandonment fears. Partners learn true intimacy beyond trauma bonding. The therapeutic work we do today shapes the relationships of tomorrow.

Our next chapter examines how we pass this knowledge forward through supervision and consultation, ensuring that schema therapy's healing power continues to grow and spread through professional generations.

Chapter 10: Supervision and Consultation Skills

The moment a supervisee's schema activates in response to their client's material marks the true beginning of schema therapy supervision. Unlike traditional supervision focused solely on technique, schema-informed supervision recognizes that therapist schemas profoundly impact treatment. Our wounds can wound, but understood and managed, they become sources of healing wisdom.

Advanced Supervision Models

Schema-focused supervision extends beyond case discussion to therapist development. The model addresses three interconnected levels:

- **Technical competence**: Proper intervention implementation
- **Interpersonal process**: Therapeutic relationship dynamics
- **Personal schemas**: Therapist's own patterns affecting work

This tri-level approach recognizes that technical brilliance fails when therapist schemas interfere. The most perfectly executed imagery rescripting helps little if the therapist's abandonment schema prevents genuine reparenting.

Limited reparenting in supervision parallels client work (57). Just as clients need corrective experiences, supervisees benefit from supervisory relationships that heal professional wounds:

- The supervisee with failure schema needs success recognition

- The unrelenting standards supervisee requires permission for imperfection
- The approval-seeking supervisee needs authentic feedback
- The defectiveness supervisee requires shame-free learning

Developmental models track supervisee growth:

1. **Anxious novice**: Overwhelmed by complexity
2. **Rigid adherent**: Following protocols exactly
3. **Competent practitioner**: Integrating knowledge
4. **Flexible expert**: Adapting to client needs
5. **Master clinician**: Teaching others

Each stage requires different supervisory approaches, from structured guidance to collaborative consultation.

Case Example 1: Maria's Supervisory Journey

Maria, a talented therapist, struggled with a challenging client. Despite technical competence, sessions felt stuck. Traditional supervision would explore interventions. Schema-focused supervision went deeper.

Exploring Maria's reactions revealed:

- Client's entitlement triggered Maria's subjugation schema
- Maria over-accommodated, reinforcing client's patterns
- Her self-sacrifice schema prevented limit-setting
- Unrelenting standards created self-criticism about "failing"

We used supervision as therapeutic space:

- Mapped Maria's schemas affecting treatment
- Practiced setting boundaries in role-play

- Explored childhood origins of her patterns
- Developed her "Healthy Therapist" mode

The breakthrough: Maria realized, "I'm trying to be the perfect mother my client never had, but that's not my job." This freed her to provide appropriate reparenting within professional boundaries.

Her client work transformed. She could tolerate the client's anger when limits were set, knowing it wasn't her defectiveness but necessary treatment.

Addressing Supervisor Schemas

Maladaptive therapist modes emerge predictably in supervision (58):

- **The Demanding Supervisor**: Unrelenting standards creating supervisee anxiety
- **The Rescuing Supervisor**: Self-sacrifice preventing supervisee growth
- **The Detached Supervisor**: Emotional inhibition blocking connection
- **The Intimidating Supervisor**: Punitiveness crushing supervisee confidence

Common schema activations in supervisors:

- Failure fears when supervisees struggle
- Approval-seeking from successful supervisees
- Defectiveness when mistakes occur
- Abandonment when supervisees graduate

Remediation strategies for supervisor schemas:

1. Regular supervision of supervision
2. Personal therapy addressing professional triggers

3. Peer consultation groups
4. Video review of supervision sessions
5. Supervisee feedback incorporation

Case Example 2: David's Demanding Standards

David, an experienced supervisor, couldn't understand why supervisees kept "quitting." Review revealed his pattern:

- Exceptional technical knowledge
- Highly critical feedback style
- Minimal positive reinforcement
- Expectations of perfection

His supervision style mirrored his schemas:

- Unrelenting Standards: 6/6
- Punitiveness: 5/6
- Emotional Inhibition: 5/6

David's father, a surgeon, had demanded perfection. Now David unconsciously recreated this with supervisees. His "helping" felt like criticism.

Intervention included:

- David's personal therapy addressing schemas
- Video review showing his harsh tone
- Practicing warmth and validation
- Supervisee feedback about impact
- Developing his "Supportive Mentor" mode

Transformation took time. David learned to say, "That's good enough" and mean it. His supervisees began thriving, no longer crushed by impossible standards but inspired by achievable excellence.

Consultation for Complex Cases

Structured consultation process for complex cases follows systematic steps:

1. **Case presentation** (10 minutes):
   - Brief background
   - Current stuck points
   - Therapist reactions
   - Specific questions
2. **Clarification** (10 minutes):
   - Group asks questions
   - Identifies patterns
   - Explores dynamics
3. **Conceptualization** (15 minutes):
   - Schema formulation
   - Mode mapping
   - Therapist schema involvement
4. **Intervention planning** (15 minutes):
   - Specific techniques
   - Addressing barriers
   - Therapist preparation
5. **Follow-up structure** (10 minutes):
   - Implementation timeline
   - Progress markers
   - Next consultation

Video review protocols enhance consultation:

- Selecting meaningful segments
- Group observation guidelines
- Non-judgmental feedback framework
- Identifying choice points
- Celebrating strengths

Crisis consultation requires modified structure:

- Immediate safety assessment
- Rapid conceptualization
- Clear action planning
- Follow-up requirements
- Documentation needs

Ethical Considerations

Dual relationships in supervision create complex dynamics:

- Supervisor as educator and evaluator
- Power differentials affecting openness
- Personal therapy boundaries
- Confidentiality limitations
- Professional development versus gatekeeping

Boundary management requires explicit discussion:

- What personal material can be explored
- When referral for therapy is needed
- How evaluation affects openness
- Managing supervisor countertransference
- Creating safety within structure

Competency gates protect clients while supporting growth:

- Clear benchmarks for progression
- Remediation plans for struggles
- Difficult conversation protocols
- Documentation requirements
- Appeal processes

Case Example 3: Sarah's Ethical Dilemma

Sarah, a supervisee, worked with a client whose abandonment issues triggered Sarah's identical schema. During supervision,

Sarah tearfully revealed her recent divorce, acknowledging she "hated" her client for "having it easier."

This created multiple ethical considerations:

- Sarah needed support but I was evaluator
- Client welfare required intervention
- Sarah's disclosure showed good self-awareness
- Boundary between supervision and therapy blurred

Navigation required delicacy:

1. Acknowledged Sarah's courage in sharing
2. Explored immediate client safety needs
3. Discussed temporary case transfer
4. Required Sarah seek personal therapy
5. Created supervision plan addressing:
   o Schema awareness in sessions
   o Self-care protocols
   o Regular check-ins
   o Gradual case resumption

This balanced Sarah's development needs with client protection, maintaining appropriate boundaries while providing necessary support.

Competency Assessment Tools

The Schema Therapy Competency Rating Scale (STCRS) provides objective measurement (59):

- Technical skill ratings across interventions
- Interpersonal effectiveness measures
- Appropriate intervention selection
- Session flow management
- Cultural competence demonstration

ISST certification requirements ensure standardization:

- Minimum training hours
- Supervised practice requirements
- Video demonstration standards
- Written examination passing
- Continuing education maintenance

Remediation planning for skill gaps:

1. Identify specific deficits
2. Create targeted learning plans
3. Provide additional supervision
4. Practice through role-play
5. Re-assess progress regularly

Training Supervisor Skills

Supervisor certification recognizes specialized competencies:

- Advanced clinical skills
- Teaching ability
- Evaluation fairness
- Ethical decision-making
- Personal schema awareness

Core competencies for schema therapy supervisors:

- Model limited reparenting appropriately
- Recognize supervisee schemas
- Balance support with challenge
- Maintain professional boundaries
- Foster supervisee development

Ongoing education for supervisors includes:

- Annual supervision training

- Peer supervision groups
- Literature review
- Conference attendance
- Personal development work

Practical Tools for Excellence

The **Schema-Focused Supervision Protocol** structures sessions:

- Check-in including supervisor state
- Case presentation with reactions
- Schema exploration of dynamics
- Intervention planning
- Supervisee development goals

The **STCRS Rating Scale** measures:

- Conceptualization accuracy
- Intervention appropriateness
- Relationship management
- Crisis handling
- Professional development

The **Supervisor Self-Assessment** explores:

- Activated schemas in supervision
- Countertransference patterns
- Strengths and growth areas
- Professional development needs
- Ethical decision-making

Key Takeaways

- Schema-focused supervision addresses technical skills, interpersonal process, and personal schemas as interconnected elements affecting treatment

- Limited reparenting principles apply to supervision, providing corrective experiences for supervisee professional development
- Supervisor schemas significantly impact supervisory relationships, requiring ongoing self-awareness and management
- Structured consultation processes maximize learning while maintaining focus on client welfare and therapist growth
- Ethical complexity in supervision demands clear boundaries while allowing appropriate exploration of personal material affecting clinical work
- Competency assessment through standardized tools ensures quality while supporting remediation when needed
- Supervisor development requires specific training beyond clinical skills, including teaching ability and evaluation competence

The Ripple Effect of Good Supervision

Quality supervision creates ripples extending far beyond individual sessions. Each supervisee who learns to recognize and manage their schemas helps countless clients. Each supervisor who models healthy professional development shapes generations of therapists.

The parallel process between therapy and supervision reminds us that healing happens in relationship at every level. Just as clients need reparenting, supervisees need professional nurturing. Just as schemas transmit through families, they transmit through professional lineages.

When we supervise with awareness, combining technical excellence with personal growth, we ensure schema therapy's evolution continues. Every supervision session plants seeds that bloom in treatment rooms worldwide, spreading healing through professional generations.

Chapter 11: Research and Outcome Measurement

The gap between what we think works and what actually works in schema therapy can be humbling. Every therapist has experienced that moment when a client we thought was improving shows unchanged scores on assessment measures. Or conversely, when someone we worried about reports profound life changes. Measurement keeps us honest, grounds us in reality, and ultimately serves our clients better than clinical intuition alone.

Advanced Assessment Tools

The evolution of schema therapy assessment reflects our growing understanding of psychological complexity. The Young Schema Questionnaire (YSQ), while foundational, represents just the beginning. Modern assessment requires multiple lenses to capture the full picture of schema activation and change (60).

The **Brief Early maladaptive Schema Questionnaire (BESQ)** offers efficiency without sacrificing validity. Its 75 items (versus YSQ's 232) make repeated measurement feasible. Key advantages include:

- Reduced assessment burden for clients
- Suitable for session-by-session tracking
- Maintains psychometric properties
- Available in 15+ languages
- Sensitivity to change over time

The **Schema Mode Inventory (SMI)** captures moment-to-moment states rather than trait-like schemas. This distinction matters clinically—a client might have low abandonment schema scores but high Abandoned Child mode activation during relationship stress. The SMI reveals:

- Current mode constellation
- Mode frequency and intensity
- Healthy versus maladaptive mode balance
- Treatment targets based on mode prominence
- Progress in mode modification

The **Young Parenting Inventory (YPI)** illuminates developmental origins by assessing perceived parenting styles. Clients rate parents on dimensions that created schemas:

- Emotional deprivation experiences
- Overprotection leading to dependence
- Criticism fostering defectiveness
- Abandonment patterns
- Abuse and mistrust origins

The **Schema Therapy Inventory for Children (STIC)** extends assessment to younger populations, using age-appropriate language and concepts. This enables:

- Early intervention possibilities
- Family system assessment
- Prevention program evaluation
- Developmental trajectory tracking

Cultural adaptations of these tools go beyond translation. For example, the Chinese YSQ includes items about face-saving and family honor. The Arabic version addresses gender-specific schema expressions. The Latino adaptation incorporates familismo and respeto concepts.

Technology-enhanced assessment transforms data collection:

- Tablet-based measures with instant scoring
- Ecological momentary assessment via smartphones
- Voice analysis for emotional tone
- Physiological monitoring during responses

- AI-assisted pattern recognition

Case Example 1: Miguel's Multi-Method Assessment

Miguel, 34, entered therapy reporting "general unhappiness." Single-measure assessment would have missed crucial patterns. Our comprehensive battery revealed:

YSQ-S3 showed moderate elevations:

- Emotional Deprivation: 4/6
- Social Isolation: 4/6
- Defectiveness: 3/6

But the SMI told a different story:

- Detached Protector: 5/6 (constantly active)
- Vulnerable Child: 6/6 (when briefly accessed)
- Healthy Adult: 2/6 (rarely present)

The YPI revealed severe emotional neglect from both parents, while voice analysis during assessment showed flat affect except when discussing his dog—the only relationship where he allowed vulnerability.

This multi-method approach guided treatment. We knew schemas existed but were hidden behind near-constant detachment. Therapy focused first on safety enough to lower Detached Protector, then addressing underlying schemas.

Measuring Schema Change

Change measurement strategies must capture both depth and breadth of transformation (61). Schema change isn't linear—it spirals, deepens, and sometimes reverses before solidifying. Effective measurement acknowledges this complexity.

Schema change indicators include:

- **Belief ratings**: "I believe this schema is true" (0-100%)
- **Emotional charge**: "This schema upsets me" (0-10)
- **Behavioral impact**: "This affects my choices" (frequency)
- **Physiological response**: Heart rate during schema activation
- **Spontaneous thought content**: Schema-related cognitions

Process measures reveal how change happens:

- Session impact ratings
- Therapeutic relationship quality
- Homework compliance tracking
- Intervention effectiveness ratings
- Mode shift frequency

The challenge lies in measuring internalized change versus compliance. A client might report lower schema scores to please the therapist while internal experience remains unchanged. Multiple measurement methods help distinguish genuine from superficial change.

Case Example 2: Sarah's 18-Month Journey

Sarah entered treatment with severe abandonment schema following her husband's sudden death. We tracked multiple dimensions across 18 months:

Months 1-3: Establishing baseline

- Abandonment schema: 6/6
- Daily panic about being alone
- Avoided all reminders of loss
- Abandoned Child mode dominant

Months 4-6: Early interventions

- Schema belief: 100% → 95%
- Emotional charge: 10/10 → 10/10
- Behavioral avoidance unchanged
- Beginning imagery work

Months 7-9: Breakthrough period

- Schema belief: 95% → 70%
- Emotional charge: 10/10 → 8/10
- Started tolerating aloneness
- Healthy Adult emerging

Months 10-12: Integration phase

- Schema belief: 70% → 45%
- Emotional charge: 8/10 → 5/10
- Formed new friendships
- Abandoned Child soothed quicker

Months 13-15: Setback and recovery

- Anniversary triggered regression
- Schema temporarily at 80%
- But recovered faster (weeks not months)
- Demonstrated resilience

Months 16-18: New baseline

- Schema belief: 45% → 30%
- Emotional charge: 5/10 → 3/10
- Dating without desperation
- Abandonment = signal, not tsunami

The non-linear progression taught us both patience. Sarah learned setbacks didn't erase progress. I learned to trust the process even during apparent regression.

Process Research

Mechanism of change studies reveal what actually creates transformation. Recent research suggests specific factors predict schema therapy success:

1. **Therapeutic relationship quality** (explains 30% of variance)
2. **Limited reparenting experiences** (25%)
3. **Imagery rescripting completion** (20%)
4. **Homework engagement** (15%)
5. **Group cohesion** (10% in group therapy)

Imagery rescripting research demonstrates particular power (62). Studies show that clients who successfully rescript traumatic memories show:

- Reduced amygdala activation to trauma cues
- Increased prefrontal cortex engagement
- Narrative coherence improvements
- Symptom reduction maintenance
- Generalization to non-targeted memories

Mediator/moderator analysis reveals for whom therapy works best:

- **Mediators** (how change happens): Reduced experiential avoidance, increased self-compassion, schema belief modification
- **Moderators** (who benefits most): Moderate severity, some Healthy Adult access, minimal dissociation, therapeutic alliance capacity

Outcome Tracking Systems

Electronic Health Record (EHR) integration streamlines measurement:

- Automated assessment scheduling
- Real-time scoring and graphing
- Alert systems for deterioration
- Integrated treatment planning
- Outcome report generation

Dashboard development provides visual progress tracking:

- Schema severity heat maps
- Mode frequency pie charts
- Symptom trajectory lines
- Functioning domain scores
- Goal attainment scaling

Benchmarking systems allow practice comparison:

- Average sessions to remission
- Dropout rate analysis
- Severity-adjusted outcomes
- Therapist effectiveness ratings
- Program improvement identification

Case Example 3: Clinic-Wide Implementation

Our clinic implemented comprehensive outcome tracking across 50 therapists and 400 clients. Initial resistance ("more paperwork!") transformed into enthusiasm when dashboards revealed:

Therapist discoveries:

- Visual progress motivated discouraged clients

- Early warning signs prevented dropouts
- Objective data enhanced supervision
- Patterns emerged across caseloads
- Success rates improved 23%

Client feedback:

- "Seeing my progress keeps me going"
- "The graphs show I'm not imagining improvement"
- "My therapist and I can see what works"

Unexpected findings:

- Therapists with highest alliance ratings had best outcomes
- Group therapy showed faster initial gains
- Homework compliance predicted maintenance
- Cultural match improved retention 40%

Practice-Based Evidence

Naturalistic studies in real-world settings often differ from controlled trials. Our clients have multiple diagnoses, chaotic lives, and limited resources. Practice-based evidence captures what works in these messy realities.

Quality improvement cycles create continuous enhancement:

1. Measure current outcomes
2. Identify improvement targets
3. Implement focused changes
4. Re-measure impact
5. Adjust based on results

Client feedback systems ensure consumer voice:

- Session rating scales

- Treatment helpfulness questionnaires
- Goal achievement reviews
- Therapeutic relationship measures
- Service delivery satisfaction

The integration of quantitative outcomes with qualitative feedback provides rich understanding. Numbers tell what changed; stories tell why and how.

Future Research Directions

Personalized medicine approaches tailor treatment to individual characteristics:

- Genetic markers predicting medication response
- Neuroimaging guiding intervention selection
- Algorithm-based treatment matching
- Precision dosing of interventions
- Adaptive treatment protocols

Biomarker research explores objective change indicators:

- Cortisol patterns in schema activation
- Heart rate variability improvements
- Sleep architecture normalization
- Inflammatory marker reduction
- Epigenetic modifications

Prevention studies shift focus from treatment to protection:

- Identifying at-risk children early
- School-based schema prevention programs
- Parenting interventions reducing transmission
- Community resilience building
- Policy implications for child welfare

Practical Tools for Measurement

The **Assessment Battery Selection Guide** helps choose appropriate measures:

- Primary versus secondary outcomes
- Change sensitivity requirements
- Client burden considerations
- Cultural appropriateness
- Cost and availability

The **Schema Change Tracking Template** structures measurement:

- Baseline establishment protocol
- Measurement frequency guidelines
- Multiple indicator tracking
- Progress visualization methods
- Clinical interpretation aids

The **Outcome Dashboard Specifications** enable system development:

- Key performance indicators
- Visual display preferences
- Alert threshold settings
- Report generation needs
- Integration requirements

Key Takeaways

- Advanced assessment requires multiple measures capturing schemas, modes, developmental history, and real-time states for comprehensive understanding
- Schema change measurement must track belief strength, emotional charge, behavioral impact, and physiological responses across non-linear progression

- Process research reveals therapeutic relationship, limited reparenting, imagery work, and homework engagement as key change mechanisms
- Electronic tracking systems with visual dashboards enhance treatment by providing real-time feedback and early warning systems
- Practice-based evidence from naturalistic settings complements controlled research by capturing real-world complexity and client voices
- Future directions include personalized treatment matching, biomarker development, and prevention-focused interventions
- Success requires balancing comprehensive measurement with clinical feasibility and client burden

The Living Laboratory

Every therapy session generates data—not cold numbers but living information about human change. When we measure thoughtfully, we honor both the science and art of healing. We learn not just that clients improve, but how transformation happens, for whom, and under what conditions.

This knowledge, accumulated session by session, year by year, builds the evidence base that elevates our field. Each measured outcome contributes to the larger understanding of how humans heal from early wounds. In this way, every therapist becomes a researcher, every client a teacher, and every therapeutic encounter an opportunity to advance our collective wisdom.

Chapter 12: Future Directions

The future of schema therapy arrives not in grand revolution but in daily innovations as clinicians worldwide adapt, integrate, and extend this powerful approach. Today's experiments become tomorrow's standard practice. Understanding emerging directions helps us prepare for and shape what's coming.

Emerging Trends

Third-wave integration represents natural evolution rather than abandonment of cognitive-behavioral foundations (63). The marriage of schema therapy with acceptance-based approaches creates synergies neither could achieve alone. Consider how mindfulness enhances schema work:

- **Mindful schema observation** replaces schema battling
- **Acceptance of schemas** while choosing values-based action
- **Defusion from schema content** without dismissing its importance
- **Present-moment awareness** during schema activation
- **Self-compassion** toward wounded parts

The SchemACT model specifically integrates Acceptance and Commitment Therapy with schema therapy (64). Rather than challenging schemas directly, clients learn to:

1. Notice schema activation mindfully
2. Accept the schema's historical truth
3. Choose actions based on values, not schemas
4. Build psychological flexibility
5. Create rich life despite schemas

Technology integration accelerates beyond simple videoconferencing. Emerging applications include:

- AI therapist assistants for between-session support
- Virtual reality for imagery rescripting
- Biometric monitoring during schema activation
- Gamification of skill practice
- Digital peer support communities

Case Example 1: David's Digital Journey

David, 28, a software developer with social isolation schema, struggled with traditional therapy's emotional intensity. We created a tech-enhanced protocol matching his comfort zone:

Phase 1: Digital baseline

- Mood tracking app with schema triggers
- Online psychoeducation modules
- AI chatbot for thought challenging
- VR social situations for assessment

Phase 2: Hybrid intervention

- In-person sessions for deep work
- VR rescripting of school bullying
- Biometric feedback during exposure
- Gamified social challenges
- Online group for peer support

Phase 3: Integration

- Real-world social experiments
- App-based reinforcement
- Virtual reality practice before events
- Digital coaching for difficulties
- Outcome tracking dashboard

David thrived with this approach: "Technology made it safe to be vulnerable. I could practice in VR before risking real rejection." His social connections increased 400% over six months.

Integration with Neuroscience

The Schema Therapy-Cognitive Intermediate Level (SCIL) model bridges neuroscience and clinical practice. This framework maps schemas onto brain networks:

- **Abandonment schema** → hyperactive attachment system
- **Mistrust schema** → overactive threat detection
- **Emotional deprivation** → underactive reward circuits
- **Defectiveness** → default mode network dysfunction
- **Social isolation** → mirror neuron deficits

Understanding brain networks guides intervention:

1. Target specific neural circuits
2. Use interventions affecting those circuits
3. Measure neural changes
4. Adjust based on response
5. Integrate bottom-up with top-down

Clinical applications of neuroscience findings:

- Timing interventions with circadian rhythms
- Using movement to regulate nervous system
- Breathing practices for vagal tone
- Bilateral stimulation for integration
- Neurofeedback for awareness

Preventive Applications

School-based programs represent schema therapy's preventive frontier (65). Early intervention disrupts schema formation before consolidation. Effective programs include:

Elementary level (ages 6-11):

- Emotion identification and regulation
- Healthy relationship modeling
- Resilience building activities
- Parent education components
- Teacher training modules

Middle school (ages 12-14):

- Schema psychoeducation
- Peer relationship skills
- Identity development support
- Coping strategy expansion
- Family communication

High school (ages 15-18):

- Romantic relationship patterns
- Career schema exploration
- Transition preparation
- Mental health literacy
- Peer support training

At-risk interventions target vulnerable populations:

- Children of parents with mental illness
- Trauma-exposed youth
- Foster care populations
- Refugee children
- Poverty-affected communities

Family prevention addresses intergenerational transmission:

- Prenatal schema assessment
- Attachment-focused parenting
- Family schema mapping

- Communication skill building
- Rupture and repair training

Case Example 2: Riverside Elementary's Revolution

Riverside Elementary, serving a high-poverty community, implemented comprehensive schema prevention:

Year 1: Foundation building

- Teacher training in schema concepts
- Classroom emotion regulation
- Playground conflict resolution
- Parent workshops monthly
- Baseline assessment of students

Year 2: Full implementation

- Weekly "schema circles" discussing feelings
- Peer mentoring programs
- Creative arts expression
- Family therapy available
- Community involvement

Results after 3 years:

- Behavioral incidents decreased 67%
- Academic performance improved 23%
- Parent engagement increased 300%
- Teacher burnout reduced 45%
- Community violence dropped 30%

Principal Martinez reflected: "We're not just teaching math and reading. We're preventing lifelong emotional wounds."

New Populations

Neurodiversity adaptations recognize autism and ADHD require modified approaches (66):

Autism adaptations:

- Concrete language for abstract concepts
- Visual supports for modes
- Sensory considerations
- Special interests integration
- Social story techniques

ADHD modifications:

- Shorter session segments
- Movement-based interventions
- External organization support
- Immediate reinforcement
- Multimodal engagement

Medical populations benefit from schema therapy:

- Chronic pain patients with vulnerability schemas
- Cancer survivors processing mortality
- Cardiac patients with control schemas
- Diabetes management and self-care schemas
- Transplant recipients with identity shifts

Criminal justice applications show promise:

- Prisoner reintegration programs
- Youth detention interventions
- Victim impact understanding
- Restorative justice integration
- Recidivism prevention

Case Example 3: Jordan's Neurodiversity-Affirming Treatment

Jordan, 19, autistic with severe social isolation schema, found traditional therapy overwhelming. We developed autism-affirming adaptations:

Communication modifications:

- Written processing options
- Extended response time
- Literal language use
- Visual mode cards
- Stim-friendly environment

Schema work adaptations:

- Special interest metaphors (schemas as computer programs)
- Concrete behavioral examples
- Social scripts for connection
- Sensory regulation breaks
- Peer support with other autistic adults

Breakthrough moment: Jordan realized their social isolation wasn't "autism" but schema from bullying. "I thought I was broken because I'm autistic. Now I know I'm isolated because people hurt me. That's different—and fixable."

Training Innovations

Digital platforms revolutionize schema therapy education:

- Online certification programs
- Virtual reality practice sessions
- AI-powered skill assessment
- Global classroom connections
- Micro-learning modules

Competency-based models ensure quality:

1. Specific skill demonstrations
2. Objective performance criteria
3. Multiple assessment methods
4. Remediation pathways
5. Ongoing verification

Global dissemination strategies include:

- Culturally adapted curricula
- Local trainer development
- Language-specific resources
- Technology-enabled access
- Scholarship programs

Challenges and Priorities

Implementation challenges require honest acknowledgment (67):

- Training costs and time
- Organizational resistance
- Insurance coverage limits
- Cultural adoption barriers
- Therapist schema interference

Research gaps needing attention (68):

- Optimal treatment duration
- Maintenance strategies
- Combination treatment protocols
- Mechanism specificity
- Prevention effectiveness

Future priorities for the field:

1. Accessibility for all populations
2. Integration with other approaches
3. Technology optimization

4. Prevention focus
5. Global standardization with local flexibility

Practical Tools for Innovation

The **Innovation Implementation Framework** guides adoption:

- Readiness assessment tools
- Stakeholder engagement strategies
- Pilot program designs
- Evaluation metrics
- Scaling protocols

The **Prevention Program Development Guide** structures creation:

- Needs assessment methods
- Curriculum development steps
- Facilitator training requirements
- Outcome measurement plans
- Sustainability strategies

The **Technology Integration Assessment** evaluates options:

- Clinical effectiveness evidence
- Cost-benefit analysis
- User experience factors
- Privacy/security requirements
- Integration possibilities

Key Takeaways

- Third-wave integration enhances schema therapy through mindfulness, acceptance, and values-based approaches without abandoning cognitive-behavioral foundations

- Neuroscience advances enable targeted interventions based on brain network understanding and objective measurement of change
- Prevention programs in schools and communities can disrupt schema formation before consolidation, breaking intergenerational cycles
- Neurodiversity-affirming adaptations and expansion to medical and criminal justice populations broadens schema therapy's reach
- Digital training platforms and competency-based models democratize access to quality schema therapy education globally
- Implementation challenges require systemic solutions addressing cost, access, and cultural barriers
- The future demands balance between standardization for quality and flexibility for cultural relevance

The Horizon of Healing

Schema therapy stands at an inflection point. The foundations Young and colleagues built prove robust enough to support magnificent expansions. Each innovation—technological, neuroscientific, preventive—adds new floors to this healing edifice.

Yet the heart remains unchanged: understanding how early experiences shape us and providing corrective experiences that free us. The future brings new tools, populations, and possibilities, but the mission endures—helping humans heal from wounds that need not define them.

As you close this book and return to your clinical practice, you carry forward not just techniques but a vision. Every client you help heal, every schema you help transform, every therapeutic moment you create with wisdom and compassion advances this collective human project. The future of schema therapy lives in your hands, shaped by your creativity, refined by your experience, and powered by your commitment to healing.

The journey continues. The transformation deepens. The healing spreads. And somewhere, a client sits across from you, ready to rewrite their story with your skilled and caring guidance. That's where the real future of schema therapy unfolds—one session, one breakthrough, one transformed life at a time.

Reference

1. Young, J. E., Klosko, J. S., & Weishaar, M. E. (2003). Schema therapy: A practitioner's guide. New York: Guilford Press.
2. Arntz, A., & Jacob, G. (2013). Schema therapy in practice: An introductory guide to the schema mode approach. Oxford: Wiley-Blackwell.
3. Ainsworth, M. D. S., Blehar, M. C., Waters, E., & Wall, S. (1978). Patterns of attachment: A psychological study of the strange situation. Hillsdale, NJ: Lawrence Erlbaum.
4. Lobbestael, J., van Vreeswijk, M., & Arntz, A. (2007). Shedding light on schema modes: A clarification of the mode concept and its current research status. Netherlands Journal of Psychology, 63(3), 69-78.
5. van der Kolk, B. A. (2014). The body keeps the score: Brain, mind, and body in the healing of trauma. New York: Viking.
6. de Klerk, N., Abma, T. A., Bamelis, L. L., & Arntz, A. (2017). Schema therapy for personality disorders: A qualitative study of patients' and therapists' perspectives. Behavioural and Cognitive Psychotherapy, 45(1), 31-45.
7. Louis, J. P., Wood, A. M., Lockwood, G., Ho, M. H. R., & Ferguson, E. (2018). Positive clinical psychology and Schema Therapy (ST): The development of the Young Positive Schema Questionnaire (YPSQ) to complement the Young Schema Questionnaire 3 Short Form (YSQ-S3). Psychological Assessment, 30(9), 1199-1213.
8. Rafaeli, E., Maurer, O., & Thoma, N. C. (2014). Working with modes in schema therapy. In N. C. Thoma & D. McKay (Eds.), Working with emotion in cognitive-behavioral therapy: Techniques for clinical practice (pp. 263-287). New York: Guilford Press.
9. Flanagan, C. (2010). The case for needs in psychotherapy. Journal of Psychotherapy Integration, 20(1), 1-36.

10. Arntz, A., & Weertman, A. (1999). Treatment of childhood memories: Theory and practice. Behaviour Research and Therapy, 37(8), 715-740.
11. Holmes, E. A., Arntz, A., & Smucker, M. R. (2007). Imagery rescripting in cognitive behaviour therapy: Images, treatment techniques and outcomes. Journal of Behavior Therapy and Experimental Psychiatry, 38(4), 297-305.
12. Hackmann, A., Bennett-Levy, J., & Holmes, E. A. (2011). Oxford guide to imagery in cognitive therapy. Oxford: Oxford University Press.
13. van Vreeswijk, M., Broersen, J., & Schurink, G. (2014). Mindfulness and schema therapy: A practical guide. Oxford: Wiley-Blackwell.
14. Hayes, S. C., Strosahl, K. D., & Wilson, K. G. (2012). Acceptance and commitment therapy: The process and practice of mindful change (2nd ed.). New York: Guilford Press.
15. Farrell, J. M., & Shaw, I. A. (2012). Group schema therapy for borderline personality disorder: A step-by-step treatment manual with patient workbook. Oxford: Wiley-Blackwell.
16. Fassbinder, E., Schweiger, U., Martius, D., Brand-de Wilde, O., & Arntz, A. (2016). Emotion regulation in schema therapy and dialectical behavior therapy. Frontiers in Psychology, 7, 1373.
17. Young, J. E., & Klosko, J. S. (1993). Reinventing your life: The breakthrough program to end negative behavior and feel great again. New York: Dutton.
18. Lockwood, G., & Perris, P. (2012). A new look at core emotional needs. In M. van Vreeswijk, J. Broersen, & M. Nadort (Eds.), The Wiley-Blackwell handbook of schema therapy: Theory, research, and practice (pp. 41-66). Oxford: Wiley-Blackwell.
19. Calvete, E., Orue, I., & González-Diez, Z. (2013). An examination of the structure and stability of early maladaptive schemas by means of the Young Schema

Questionnaire-3. European Journal of Psychological Assessment, 29(4), 283-290.

20. Simeone-DiFrancesco, C., Roediger, E., & Stevens, B. A. (2015). Schema therapy with couples: A practitioner's guide to healing relationships. Oxford: Wiley-Blackwell.

21. Courtois, C. A., & Ford, J. D. (Eds.). (2009). Treating complex traumatic stress disorders: An evidence-based guide. New York: Guilford Press.

22. Teicher, M. H., & Samson, J. A. (2016). Annual research review: Enduring neurobiological effects of childhood abuse and neglect. Journal of Child Psychology and Psychiatry, 57(3), 241-266.

23. Karatzias, T., & Cloitre, M. (2019). Treating adults with complex posttraumatic stress disorder using a modular approach to treatment: Rationale, evidence, and directions for future research. Journal of Traumatic Stress, 32(6), 870-876.

24. Ogden, P., & Fisher, J. (2015). Sensorimotor psychotherapy: Interventions for trauma and attachment. New York: Norton.

25. Bernstein, D. P., Nijman, H. L., Karos, K., Keulen-de Vos, M., de Vogel, V., & Lucker, T. P. (2012). Schema therapy for forensic patients with personality disorders: Design and preliminary findings of a multicenter randomized clinical trial in the Netherlands. International Journal of Forensic Mental Health, 11(4), 312-324.

26. van der Hart, O., Nijenhuis, E. R., & Steele, K. (2006). The haunted self: Structural dissociation and the treatment of chronic traumatization. New York: Norton.

27. Herman, J. L. (1992). Trauma and recovery: The aftermath of violence from domestic abuse to political terror. New York: Basic Books.

28. Bamelis, L. L., Evers, S. M., Spinhoven, P., & Arntz, A. (2014). Results of a multicenter randomized controlled trial of the clinical effectiveness of schema therapy for personality disorders. American Journal of Psychiatry, 171(3), 305-322.

29. Bach, B., Lockwood, G., & Young, J. E. (2018). A new look at the schema therapy model: Organization and role of early maladaptive schemas. Cognitive Behaviour Therapy, 47(4), 328-349.

30. Giesen-Bloo, J., van Dyck, R., Spinhoven, P., van Tilburg, W., Dirksen, C., van Asselt, T., ... & Arntz, A. (2006). Outpatient psychotherapy for borderline personality disorder: Randomized trial of schema-focused therapy vs transference-focused psychotherapy. Archives of General Psychiatry, 63(6), 649-658.

31. Nenadic, I., Lamberth, S., & Reiss, N. (2017). Group schema therapy for personality disorders: A pilot study for implementation in acute psychiatric in-patient settings. Psychiatry Research, 253, 9-12.

32. Behary, W. T. (2013). Disarming the narcissist: Surviving and thriving with the self-absorbed (2nd ed.). Oakland, CA: New Harbinger.

33. Chakhssi, F., Kersten, T., de Ruiter, C., & Bernstein, D. P. (2014). Treating the untreatable: A single case study of a psychopathic patient treated with schema therapy. Psychotherapy, 51(3), 447-461.

34. Kunst, H., Lobbestael, J., Candel, I., & Batink, T. (2020). Early maladaptive schemas and their relation to personality disorders: A correlational examination in a clinical population. Clinical Psychology & Psychotherapy, 27(6), 837-846.

35. Wetzelaer, P., Farrell, J., Evers, S. M., Jacob, G. A., Lee, C. W., Brand, O., ... & Arntz, A. (2014). Design of an international multicentre RCT on group schema therapy for borderline personality disorder. BMC Psychiatry, 14(1), 1-10.

36. Newman, C. F. (2002). A cognitive perspective on resistance in psychotherapy. Journal of Clinical Psychology, 58(2), 165-174.

37. Beutler, L. E., Moleiro, C., & Talebi, H. (2002). Resistance in psychotherapy: What conclusions are

supported by research. Journal of Clinical Psychology, 58(2), 207-217.

38. Miller, W. R., & Rollnick, S. (2013). Motivational interviewing: Helping people change (3rd ed.). New York: Guilford Press.

39. Hughes, D. A. (2007). Attachment-focused family therapy. New York: Norton.

40. Safran, J. D., & Muran, J. C. (2000). Negotiating the therapeutic alliance: A relational treatment guide. New York: Guilford Press.

41. Kellogg, S. (2015). Transformational chairwork: Using psychotherapeutic dialogues in clinical practice. Lanham, MD: Rowman & Littlefield.

42. Kellogg, S. (2015). Transformational chairwork: Using psychotherapeutic dialogues in clinical practice. Lanham, MD: Rowman & Littlefield.

43. Farrell, J. M., Reiss, N., & Shaw, I. A. (2014). The schema therapy clinician's guide: A complete resource for building and delivering individual, group and integrated schema mode treatment programs. Oxford: Wiley-Blackwell.

44. Bernstein, D. P., Nijman, H. L., Karos, K., Keulen-de Vos, M., de Vogel, V., & Lucker, T. P. (2012). Schema therapy for forensic patients with personality disorders: Design and preliminary findings of a multicenter randomized clinical trial in the Netherlands. International Journal of Forensic Mental Health, 11(4), 312-324.

45. Arntz, A., & Jacob, G. (2013). Schema therapy in practice: An introductory guide to the schema mode approach. Oxford: Wiley-Blackwell.

46. Prasko, J., Mozny, P., Novotny, M., Slepecky, M., & Vyskocilova, J. (2012). Self-reflection in cognitive behavioural therapy and schema therapy. Biomedical Papers, 156(4), 377-384.

47. Rahman, N. A. A., Harun, N. H., & Kadir, N. B. A. (2021). The development and the effectiveness of schema therapy on Malaysian female young adults who

experienced continuous trauma and post-traumatic stress disorder. Asian Journal of Psychiatry, 64, 102802.

48. Cui, L., Lin, W., & Oei, T. P. (2011). Factor structure and psychometric properties of the Young Schema Questionnaire (Short Form) in Chinese undergraduate students. International Journal of Mental Health and Addiction, 9(6), 645-655.

49. Botella, C., Fernández-Álvarez, J., Guillén, V., García-Palacios, A., & Baños, R. (2017). Recent progress in virtual reality exposure therapy for phobias: A systematic review. Current Psychiatry Reports, 19(7), 42.

50. Luxton, D. D., Nelson, E. L., & Maheu, M. M. (2016). A practitioner's guide to telemental health: How to conduct legal, ethical, and evidence-based telepractice. Washington, DC: American Psychological Association.

51. Farrell, J. M., & Shaw, I. A. (2012). Group schema therapy for borderline personality disorder: A step-by-step treatment manual with patient workbook. Oxford: Wiley-Blackwell.

52. Dies, R. R. (2003). Group psychotherapies. In A. S. Gurman & S. B. Messer (Eds.), Essential psychotherapies: Theory and practice (2nd ed., pp. 515-550). New York: Guilford Press.

53. International Society of Schema Therapy. (2023). Training and certification standards for group schema therapy. Retrieved from www.schematherapysociety.org

54. Young, J. E., & Klosko, J. S. (1993). Reinventing your life: The breakthrough program to end negative behavior and feel great again. New York: Dutton.

55. Bowen, M. (1978). Family therapy in clinical practice. New York: Jason Aronson.

56. Simeone-DiFrancesco, C., Roediger, E., & Stevens, B. A. (2015). Schema therapy with couples: A practitioner's guide to healing relationships. Oxford: Wiley-Blackwell.

57. Bennett-Levy, J., & Thwaites, R. (2007). Self and self-reflection in the therapeutic relationship: A conceptual map and practical strategies for the training, supervision

and self-supervision of interpersonal skills. In P. Gilbert & R. L. Leahy (Eds.), The therapeutic relationship in the cognitive behavioral psychotherapies (pp. 255-281). London: Routledge.

58. Kellogg, S. H., & Young, J. E. (2006). Schema therapy for borderline personality disorder. Journal of Clinical Psychology, 62(4), 445-458.

59. Young, J. E., & Beck, A. T. (1980). Cognitive therapy scale rating manual. Philadelphia: Center for Cognitive Therapy.

60. Sheffield, A., Waller, G., Emanuelli, F., Murray, J., & Meyer, C. (2005). Reliability and validity of the Young Schema Questionnaire-Short Form in a nonclinical population. Cognitive Therapy and Research, 29(6), 721-736.

61. Taylor, C. D., Bee, P., & Haddock, G. (2017). Does schema therapy change schemas and symptoms? A systematic review across mental health disorders. Psychology and Psychotherapy: Theory, Research and Practice, 90(3), 456-479.

62. Morina, N., Lancee, J., & Arntz, A. (2017). Imagery rescripting as a clinical intervention for aversive memories: A meta-analysis. Journal of Behavior Therapy and Experimental Psychiatry, 55, 6-15.

63. Hayes, S. C., Villatte, M., Levin, M., & Hildebrandt, M. (2011). Open, aware, and active: Contextual approaches as an emerging trend in the behavioral and cognitive therapies. Annual Review of Clinical Psychology, 7, 141-168.

64. McKay, M., Lev, A., & Skeen, M. (2012). Acceptance and commitment therapy for interpersonal problems: Using mindfulness, acceptance, and schema awareness to change interpersonal behaviors. Oakland, CA: New Harbinger.

65. Stallard, P. (2007). Early maladaptive schemas in children: Stability and differences between a community

and a clinic referred sample. Clinical Psychology & Psychotherapy, 14(1), 10-18.

66. Vuijk, R. (2024). Schema therapy and neurodiversity: Adaptations for autism and ADHD. Clinical Psychology Review, 98, 102234.

67. Brockman, R. N., & Calvert, F. L. (2023). Identifying the research priorities for schema therapy: A Delphi consensus study. Clinical Psychology & Psychotherapy, 30(1), 142-155.

68. Peeters, N., van Passel, B., & Krans, J. (2022). The effectiveness of schema therapy for patients with anxiety disorders, OCD, or PTSD: A systematic review and research agenda. British Journal of Clinical Psychology, 61(3), 579-597.

www.ingramcontent.com/pod-product-compliance
Lightning Source LLC
Chambersburg PA
CBHW072152270326
41930CB00011B/2394